Pr
R1
"A

nurses. I particularly like the inclusion of specific questions to ask regarding each system and the step-by-step instructions to guide physical assessment. Even experienced nurses will welcome the helpful reminders included in each chapter to make their patient assessments more thorough."

AMY HADDAD, RN, PhD
Associate Dean
School of Pharmacy and Allied Health Professions
Creighton University, Omaha, Neb.

"Just what I've been looking for—a book that sifts through the 'nice to know' and focuses on what I 'need to know' at the bedside when I work in the ED. Not only will I carry this book with me for reference, but I'll also put it on the reading list for my students."

PATRICIA CARROLL, RN,C, MS, CEN, RRT
Independent Nurse Consultant
Per diem staff nurse, ED
Manchester Memorial Hospital, Manchester, Conn.

"*RN's Pocket Assessment Guide* provides assessment information and helpful hints in an easy-to-read format. Its pocket size makes it an ideal reference for the experienced nurse or for nurses interested in improving their assessment skills."

PAT SNOWBERGER, RN,C, MSN
Director, Educational Services
Trumbull Memorial Hospital, Warren, Ohio

Pocket Assessment Guide

Quick, Accurate Evaluation of Adult Acute Care Patients

Edited by
Roberta L. Messner, RN,C, PhD, CPHQ
Suzanne Wolfe

MEDICAL ECONOMICS
MONTVALE, NEW JERSEY

Library of Congress Catalog Number: 97-76611
ISBN: 1-56363-273-X
Manufactured in the United States of America

Bulk copy inquiries are invited.
Contact the Trade Sales Department at 1-800-442-6657.

The information presented in this publication is based on research and consultation with nursing experts. To the best of our knowledge, it represents current opinion at the time of publication. It cannot be construed, however, as absolute and universal recommendations or as clinical advice in any given situation. The authors, editors, and publisher disclaim responsibility for any adverse consequences that result from application of the information in this book, from undetected errors or omissions, or from misinterpretation by the reader.

RN© is a trademark of Medical Economics registered in the U.S. Patent & Trademark Office.

Copyright © 1997 and published by Medical Economics at Montvale, NJ 07645. All rights reserved. None of the content of this publication may be reproduced, stored in a retrieval system, or transmitted in any form or by any means (electronic, mechanical, photocopying, recording, or otherwise) without prior written permission of the publisher. For information, address *RN* Magazine, Five Paragon Drive, Montvale NJ 07645.

Publishing staff: Marianne Dekker Mattera, editorial director, *RN*; Terri J. Metules, RN, BSN, CCRN, clinical editor, *RN*; Paul L. Cerrato, senior editor, *RN*; Lydia Biagioli, production manager; Joanne Pearson, production associate; Robert Hartman, art director.

Cover Illustration: Kevin Somerville

Business staff: Paul Walsh, publisher; Marjorie Duffy, production director; Robin Bartlett, director, trade and direct marketing sales; Stephanie DeNardi and Steven Schweikhart, fulfillment managers.

Officers of Medical Economics: President and Chief Executive Officer: Curtis B. Allen; Vice President, Human Resources: Pamela M. Bilash; Vice President and Chief Information Officer: Steven M. Bressler; Vice President, Finance, and Chief Financial Officer: Thomas W. Ehardt; Executive Vice President and Chief Operating Officer: Rick Noble; Executive Vice President, Magazine Publishing: Thomas F. Rice; Senior Vice President, Operations: John R. Ware

About the Editors

ROBERTA L. MESSNER, RN,C, PhD, CPHQ has more than 20 years of nursing experience, including work in the areas of critical care, med/surg, gastroenterology, infection control, and quality improvement. She is currently Patient Health Education Coordinator at the Veterans Affairs Medical Center in Huntington, W. Va. A member of the *RN* Editorial Board, Dr. Messner has been listed in *Who's Who in America* and *Who's Who in American Nursing*. She is co-editor of the *Manual of Psychosocial Nursing Interventions: Promoting Mental Health in Medical-Surgical Settings* and co-author of *Increasing Patient Satisfaction: A Guide for Nurses*.

SUZANNE WOLFE is Articles Editor of *RN*, and has been shaping the editorial content of that publication since 1992. She has more than 10 years of experience editing and writing clinical and nonclinical material for nurses, physicians, and other health care professionals. Her work on *RN* has earned her a Jesse H. Neal Editorial Achievement Award—considered the Pulitzer prize of specialized journalism—and a Neal Certificate of Merit.

Contents

Contributors	IX
Preface	XI
1. Taking a history	1
2. The physical exam	11
3. Integumentary system	19
4. Head, neck, and cranial nerves	35
5. Nervous system	55
6. Respiratory system	69
7. Cardiac system	89
8. Peripheral vascular system	107
9. Gastrointestinal system	127
10. Genitourinary system	143
11. Geriatric patients: Special considerations	159

Appendices

1. Standard lab values	175
2. Interpreting ABGs	180
3. Hemodynamic parameters	182
4. Calculating drug dosages and drip rates	185
5. Medication monitoring: Therapeutic ranges and serum drug interactions	189
6. A guide to transfusing blood products	192
7. Differentiating chest pain	198
8. Shock: Signs and symptoms	202
9. Electrolyte imbalances: Signs and symptoms	204
10. Recognizing endocrine emergencies	208
11. Classifying burns	214
12. A guide to religious practices	216

Bibliography	**225**
Art/Photo Credits	**228**
Index	**229**

Contributors

GAYLE P. ANDRESEN, RN,C, MS, ANP/GNP
Consultant in gerontologic nursing
Formerly, Senior Instructor in Family Medicine
University of Colorado, Denver
Geriatric patients

ELLEN BARKER, RN, MSN, CNRN
Neuroscience Clinical Specialist
Neuroscience Nursing Consultants
Greenville, Del.
Head, neck, and cranial nerves
Nervous system

CYNTHIA FINESILVER, RN,C, MSN, CNRN
Assistant Professor
Bellin College of Nursing
Green Bay, Wisc.
Respiratory system

MARGARET A. FITZGERALD, RN,CS, MS, FNP
President, Fitzgerald Health Education Associates
Andover, Mass.
Family Nurse Practitioner
Greater Lawrence (MA) Family Health Center
The physical exam

CHRISTY FLORY, RN,C, MS
Adult Nurse Practitioner
Department of Dermatology
Beth Israel Deaconess Medical Center
Boston, Mass.
Integumentary system

PATSY EILEEN GEHRING, RN, PhD
Assistant Professor of Nursing
Lakeland Community College
Mentor, Ohio
Taking a history
Peripheral vascular system

CINDY HOLMGREN, RN, MSN, OCN
Assistant Professor
Bellin College of Nursing
Green Bay, Wisc.
Gastrointestinal system

KATHLEEN A. MOORE, RN, BS, CCRN
Formerly, Clinical Editor of *RN* and Staff Nurse
Neuro Intensive Care
Columbia-Presbyterian Medical Center
New York, N.Y.
Head, neck, and cranial nerves
Nervous system

JOANNE J. TATE, RN, BSN, MEd, MNAD/MNED, PhD
Teaching Specialist
Shadyside Hospital School of Nursing
Pittsburgh, Penn.
Genitourinary system

LINDA YACONE-MORTON, RN, BS, CCRN
Clinical Nurse
Intermediate Cardiac Care Unit
Thomas Jefferson University Hospital
Philadelphia, Penn.
Cardiac system

Preface

Physical assessment, like much of nursing, is both science and art. To determine if the liver is enlarged, you need not only facts—like where the liver is located in the abdomen and how to palpate properly—you need a feel for how deeply to press and a memory of what a liver feels like when your fingers approach it through layers of skin and muscle.

You learned the facts and at least some of the feeling in school. You build memory through years of practice. You refine your art constantly. In this book, we hope to help you in that continuous process. Here, expert nurses tell you what your system review should cover, what questions to ask to elicit an accurate history, and where and how to look, listen, and palpate. They explain what's normal and what's not, and give examples of conditions that your assessment findings point to. Rounding out this information are a dozen appendices that will serve as quick reference tools in a host of situations.

For new nurses, this book can help hone technique and promote confidence. For experienced nurses, it can serve as an extended memory bank and a bedside security blanket. For nurses who cross-train and float, it can be a professional survival guide to working on another unit. Wherever you care for patients and for however long you have been doing it, it's our hope that making this pocket guide a part of your "walking" library will help you become a better nurse, and make one of the most demanding jobs around that much easier to do.

CHAPTER ONE

Taking a history

History. Take the word apart: his story. An appropriate term for the process through which we learn about the patient and his illness from his point of view.

The best way to get that story is to take a step-by-step approach. Generally, the history you take will be an episodic one—concentrating on the patient's current illness—rather than a birth-to-present chronicle.

Keep in mind, clinical interviewing is a *skill* that must be learned and practiced in order to obtain the best and most relevant information.

INTRODUCTIONS

- Introduce yourself, identify your position, and briefly explain the purpose of the interview.
- Do not call the patient by his first name unless he's given you permission to do so. Do not use demeaning or overly familiar terms, such as "dear" or "pops."
- Present yourself as a self-assured, competent, and respectful professional.
- Check to be sure the badge that states your name and position is clearly visible.
- Be careful that your body language does not communicate disinterest.
- Determine whether a language barrier exists and get an interpreter if necessary.
- Pull the curtains for privacy and excuse the family; you can take information from them later.
- Before starting the interview, be sure the patient is comfortable (e.g., provide a bedpan, elevate the head of the bed).
- Sit about three feet from the patient, a distance that's neither intimate nor so far away that private communication is uncomfortable.
- Lean forward and maintain eye contact.
- Tell the patient you will be making brief notes, which you'll review with him when you're finished to make sure you've understood him correctly.
- Assure him that any information he gives you will be shared only with those who need it to provide appropriate care.

With hearing impaired patients:

- Determine whether the patient has a hearing aid. If he does, check that it is turned on and working.
- If appropriate, move the patient to an area with minimal background noise.
- Speak at a normal pace.
- Look straight at the patient to facilitate communication if he reads lips.
- Find out whether the patient uses sign language and enlist the aid of an interpreter if he does.
- Pay especially close attention to nonverbal cues from the patient.
- Offer to provide a pen and paper if appropriate.

With visually impaired patients:

- Be sure to face the patient while speaking.
- Use a normal volume of voice.
- Tell the patient when you are entering or leaving the room.
- Ask for the patient's permission before you touch him.

With speech impaired and aphasic patients:

- Give the patient more time than usual to answer questions. Do not answer for him.
- Use closed questions—those that can be answered in one or two words—when possible.
- Repeat or rephrase the question if the patient doesn't understand or remember it.
- For patients who have difficulty understanding what you say (receptive aphasia), use gestures to supplement your spoken words. Remember, though, patients with *speech* problems do not need your gestures. They can hear and understand, they just can't speak.

INTERVIEW TECHNIQUES

ENCOURAGE THE PATIENT TO PROVIDE COMPLETE ANSWERS.

- Say "Go on" or nod your head every so often.
- Show interest and confirm your understanding of what the patient has told you by summarizing his account periodically. ("Now, did I understand you correctly that the pain felt like a sharp jab?")
- Gently pin him down when he's unclear. For example, ask what he meant by a "spell." Tell him you realize he's not sure how long he's had symptoms, but has it been more than a week? A month?
- Do not interrupt him when he talks.

AVOID LEADING QUESTIONS AND MEDICAL JARGON.

- Rather than asking a patient with GI bleeding whether his stools look like tar, ask "What color is your stool?"
- Do not automatically assume the patient has the same medical problem that he had last time.
- Remember that even patients with a high literacy level may not understand medical terminology.

AVOID MAKING THE PATIENT FEEL GUILTY.

- Do not tell him "Patients with your problem should not have this much pain."
- Avoid "why" questions such as "Why didn't you take your pills?" or "Why didn't you come in sooner?"

SAVE SENSITIVE TOPICS FOR THE END OF THE INTERVIEW.

- Defer subjects such as the use of tobacco, alcohol, or other drugs until you and your patient have developed a rapport.
- Use the same tone of voice as with previous questions.
- Don't be embarrassed to ask detailed questions that require the patient to be specific. To probe a patient's use of alcohol, for instance, ask how much he drinks a day. Don't settle

for "I'm a social drinker." (Many clinicians use the CAGE questionnaire: Have you felt the need to **C**ut down on alcohol intake? Do you become **A**nnoyed when others comment on your intake? Do you feel **G**uilty about using alcohol? Have you ever taken an **E**ye-opener—that is, used alcohol to alleviate a hangover?)

- Maintain a nonjudgmental attitude when dealing with behaviors and beliefs that are in conflict with your own values.

USE SPECIAL APPROACHES WITH CERTAIN PATIENT POPULATIONS.

With psychiatric patients:

- A patient who answers "Yes" to all questions or makes nonsensical statements like "My hands are getting bigger" may have a mental disorder. Focus on his behavior and note his exact words.

With terminally ill patients:

- These patients often just want a sympathetic ear. Let the patient take the lead; he may want to talk about other issues.

With hostile patients:

- If possible, interview the patient in an open area with security guards nearby.
- Try to calm the patient down by offering juice or water if appropriate.
- Don't challenge the patient or register disapproval.
- If you are in a room or enclosed area, position yourself so that the patient is not between you and the door or exit. Do not close the room door.
- Don't turn your back on the patient or permit him to walk behind you.
- Be alert for signs of escalating tension, such as clenched fists and a loud, angry voice. Remove yourself from a threatening situation and call for help.

THE PATIENT PROFILE

Object: To learn anything that could have an impact on symptoms and how the patient adapts to disease. To learn how the patient best copes with health care interactions.

Cover these areas:

BIOGRAPHICAL DATA

- Age
- Occupation
- Education/literacy level
- Religion
- Hobbies
- Marital status or other intimate relationships
- Race

CULTURAL DATA

Language barriers and communication styles:

- In what language do you prefer to communicate? Do you need an interpreter?
- Are there certain ways of showing respect in your culture?
- Are there any special customs we should be aware of in regard to touching, social distance, eye contact, or other aspects of communicating?

Health beliefs and practices:

- Which member of your family is primarily responsible for making health care decisions?
- Who should we teach how to handle your particular health problems?
- Are there any cultural, religious, or ethnic practices that you want to follow (e.g., dietary restrictions, prohibitions against certain treatments)?

For a look at different religious beliefs, see Appendix 12, "A guide to religious practices."

Role of the family:

- To whom in the family or social structure should we turn for direction or communication?

PSYCHOSOCIAL DATA

Home environment:

- What type of dwelling do you live in?
- How many rooms and floors does it have?
- How many people do you live with? How old are they?

Financial resources:

- Would you require financial assistance if you were ill for any period of time?

Patient's coping mechanisms:

- How have you responded to illness and stress in the past?

Barriers to learning (e.g., physical, cognitive, emotional):

- Do you have special learning needs?

DEFINING THE CHIEF COMPLAINT

USE THE PQRST MNEMONIC

P IS FOR WHAT PROVOKES THE COMPLAINT AND FOR PALLIATIVE MEASURES.	What causes the symptom? What aggravates or alleviates it? For example, does the leg hurt while walking but feel better with rest? Has any medication or treatment worked in the past?
Q IS FOR QUALITY.	What does it feel like? (If the patient can't find words, offer suggestions: "Does the pain ache, burn, or sting?")
R IS FOR REGION (LOCATION) AND RADIATION.	Where does the symptom occur? Is it localized or diffuse? Where does it spread to? Where does it hurt most?
S IS FOR SEVERITY.	On a scale of one to 10, with 10 being the most severe, how bad is it?
T IS FOR TIMING.	When did it start? Is it continuous or intermittent?

NOTE: If the patient has several symptoms that occur together—e.g., nausea, vomiting, and abdominal pain—list them all as the chief complaint.

SYSTEM REVIEW

Probe further based on the chief complaint. For a listing of topics that should be covered for each particular body system, see the appropriate chapter.

PAST HISTORY

Obtaining details of the patient's personal health history will allow you to link the current illness with previous illnesses or injuries. Inquire about the following:

- Tests
- Surgeries
- Previous hospitalizations
- Past symptoms
- Chronic illness
- Medications (prescription and over-the-counter)
- Childhood diseases
- Allergies/allergic reactions to food or drugs
- Physical injuries
- Fever
- Diet
- Usual weight
- Change in weight/weight loss without dieting
- Weakness
- Fatigue
- Sweats
- Hot or cold intolerance
- History of anemia
- Bleeding tendencies
- Blood transfusion and possible reactions
- Exposure to radiation

FAMILY HISTORY

Obtaining a family history will allow you to determine if heredity plays a part in the patient's chief complaint. Ask about the health of blood relatives only. If you suspect an infectious disorder, however, get details about all close contacts, as well as recent travel.

CLOSING THE INTERVIEW

When your history-taking is over, ask the patient if there is anything else he would like to tell you. Assure him that you will check back later to see if other important information has occurred to him.

CHAPTER TWO

The physical exam

It's just as essential to have a system when conducting a physical exam as when taking a history. Besides helping you collect and organize information relating to the patient's chief complaint, a systematic approach that progresses through inspection, palpation, percussion, and auscultation will ensure that you don't overlook obvious signs of trouble. Following is a quick review of basic skills.

INSPECTION

Because we are always observing patients and acting on the information those observations give us, inspection is an assessment skill that we seldom think about. Although it is the part of the physical that comes first—before you touch or listen—it's often not a separate step at all. It can be accomplished while taking the initial history, for example, or when you give a patient his meds or provide a bedpan.

An organized inspection proceeds from head to toe. You observe any general characteristics first, then focus on specifics. Your initial general inspection should cover the following areas:

OVERALL APPEARANCE

- Does the patient appear acutely ill or generally well?
- What is his level of consciousness?
- Is he unkempt or well-groomed?
- Is he dressed appropriately for the weather and occasion?
- Does he look his stated age? Older? Younger?
- Is his skin color altered as a result of jaundice, cyanosis, or pallor?
- Is there any edema?
- Is his speech clear and coherent and does it flow easily? Is he able to respond to questions quickly and provide a complete history?

NUTRITIONAL STATUS

- Has the patient lost subcutaneous fat in the waist, arms, and legs?
- Has he lost muscle mass?
- Are there signs of atrophy on the arms and legs?
- Does he have rough, dry, flaky skin? Ridged nail beds? Dull hair that can be easily plucked?
- Is he obese? (May be the result of a disease such as Cushing's syndrome or chronic steroid therapy.)

POSTURE AND GAIT

- What is the patient's position on the bed or examination table? (A tripod posture—patient is propped up on elbows or palms and leaning forward—may suggest chronic obstructive pulmonary disease or acute asthma. A slumped posture may suggest depression.)
- When the patient walks, is there any shuffling, foot dragging, or a limp—possible signs of an orthopedic or neurological disorder?
- Is there any paralysis or tremor?
- Is his body movement restricted, possibly indicating pain?

SYMMETRY

- Are body parts the same size and shape? (Marked asymmetry, especially in paired organs and lymph nodes, is abnormal. Minor size differences—frequently seen in feet or breasts, for example—can be normal.)

INDIVIDUAL BODY SYSTEMS

Specifics for each system are discussed in the appropriate chapter.

Assessment approach:

Body:	Head to toe, medial to lateral, front to back
Orifices:	Outside to inside

TIPS

- Use good lighting.
- Room temperature should be comfortable; both heat and cold can affect skin color.

PALPATION

Before touching a patient, make sure your hands are not only clean but warm. Always wear gloves when examining broken or irritated skin and mucous membranes.

Start with an area that you expect to be normal, to develop a baseline for comparison. Then move on to possible trouble spots, comparing one side of the body with the other when appropriate. Have the patient take slow, deep breaths through the mouth to decrease muscle tension.

Light Palpation

HOW TO DO IT:

Keep two or three fingers together and press the skin gently with the tips to a depth of about 1/2 to 3/4 inch (approximately 1–2 cm). To check for a breast nodule, work the fingertips in a circular motion.

WHAT IT DETECTS:

Structures and masses within and directly below the skin.

Tenderness, such as that caused by soft tissue injury.

Temperature changes, such as the abnormal warmth of an arthritic joint. (Many practitioners prefer to assess temperature with the back of the hand.)

Pulmonary disorders, such as pneumonia (see Chapter 6, Respiratory System).

Deep Palpation

HOW TO DO IT:

Put one hand on top of the other and press down with the fingertips of both hands about two inches (5 cm). This maneuver traps an organ beneath the examining hand.

WHAT IT DETECTS:

Organs, masses, and tenderness within a body cavity—most commonly, the abdomen and pelvis.

FIGURE 2-1. LIGHT PALPATION.

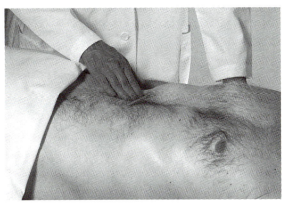

FIGURE 2-2. DEEP PALPATION.

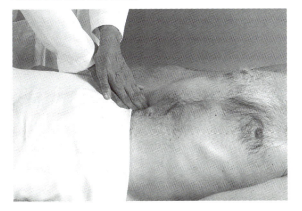

16 RN'S POCKET ASSESSMENT GUIDE

FIGURE 2-3. PERCUSSION.

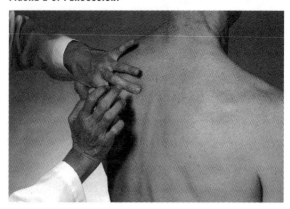

FIGURE 2-4. AUSCULTATION.

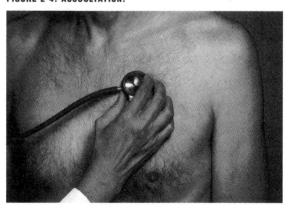

PERCUSSION

Palpation will tell you about an organ's size and location. Percussion will let you evaluate the density of underlying tissue.

HOW TO DO IT:

Place the middle finger of your left hand on the patient's body and briskly tap it with the tip of the middle finger of your right hand. (If you are left-handed, do the reverse.)

The larger a vibrating body, the more sound it makes. Thus someone with small hands may not generate enough sound with this technique. An alternative is to place your middle finger on the area and briskly strike it with the side of the thumb.

WHAT TO LISTEN FOR:

FLATNESS	A soft, high-pitched, short sound. Normally heard over bone or muscle.
RESONANCE	A loud, long, low-pitched sound. Normally heard when percussing the lungs.
HYPERRESONANCE	A loud, very long sound, lower-pitched than resonance. Lungs that are overinflated by air trapping will be hyperresonant.
DULLNESS	A medium-pitched sound of medium duration, slightly louder than the flat note generated by bone or muscle. Normal when heard over the liver. Dullness over a section of the lung can indicate increased tissue density, possibly caused by pneumonia.
TYMPANY	A high-pitched, loud sound of medium duration. Often heard over a gastric air bubble.

AUSCULTATION

Normally, you will save auscultation until last. With the abdomen, however, you will auscultate before you palpate, because pressing down on the abdominal wall may alter bowel sounds.

Auscultation is the act of listening to sounds within the body. Note pitch, intensity, duration, and quality (e.g., whistling, snapping, swooshing, gurgling). For information on specific sounds—breath, heart, vascular, and bowel—see the chapter for the corresponding system.

PROPER EQUIPMENT:

- To minimize sound distortion, stethoscope tubing should ideally be no more than 14 inches long.
- Ear pieces should fit snugly. If you can understand someone talking in the same room, they're too loose.
- Stethoscope should have a diaphragm and a bell. Use the diaphragm for higher-pitched sounds, including S_1 and S_2 heart sounds and friction rubs, and sounds heard over the lungs and abdomen. Place it firmly on the skin to block out extraneous noises.
- Use the bell to assess low-pitched sounds, including S_3 and S_4 heart sounds and certain heart murmurs. Place it lightly on the chest so that you don't push skin tissue up into the bell, causing distortion.

CHAPTER THREE

Integumentary system

Over the course of a lifetime, a person's skin is assaulted by pathogens, allergens, ultraviolet radiation, and a variety of other noxious agents. A thorough skin examination helps pinpoint many of the diseases that result if these agents penetrate the skin's defenses. It also alerts you to problems that arise from within— heart disease, for example, or blood disorders.

Recognizing such conditions as skin cancer, impetigo, scabies, and hives requires both a discriminating eye and a careful history. For color photos of common skin disorders, see pages 29-32.

SYSTEM REVIEW SHOULD COVER:

- Rashes
- Itching
- Hives
- Bruising
- History of eczema
- Dryness
- Changes in skin color
- Changes in hair texture
- Changes in nail texture
- Changes in nail appearance
- History of previous skin disorders
- Lumps
- Use of hair dyes

SPECIFIC QUESTIONS TO ASK:

- Have you had any recent skin lesions or rashes? When did they first appear? How long did they remain?
- Can they be linked to heat, cold, stress, occupation or avocational exposure to toxic material, travel to other locales, new clothing, detergents, or skin care products?
- Have you ever had any drug allergies that have caused rashes or hives?
- Do you or a family member have asthma, hay fever, or atopic dermatitis?
- Are you experiencing any pain, itching, tingling, or burning?
- Has any area of skin recently changed color?
- How much time do you spend in the sun? Do you use sunscreen?
- Have you or a family member ever had malignant melanoma or another skin cancer?

INTEGUMENTARY SYSTEM **21**

PREPARING FOR THE SKIN SURVEY

Have the patient disrobe so that you can inspect the entire epithelial surface—including the scalp, ears, mucous membranes, palms, soles, genitals, buttocks, and areas between the toes. You can preserve his privacy by allowing him to keep his underwear on until the end of the exam.

Be sure to wear gloves when examining lesions, mucous membranes, and any area that is itching—the condition may be contagious.

What you'll need:

- Adequate overhead lighting
- Penlight to examine the inside of the mouth and view elevated skin lesions from the side
- Gloves
- Ruler (mm/cm)

ASSESSING COLOR

The color of the skin or the lack of it not only points to certain topical problems, but can tip you off to underlying systemic conditions. Because people of different races or ethnic backgrounds have different skin tones, remember while doing your exam that you are looking for changes in the patient's normal skin color.

What you'll look for:
Skin that's unusually pale or dark

ASSESSMENT FINDING	WHAT IT CAN MEAN
PALE	
Patches of hypopigmentation:	
Especially on the chest, upper back, and neck	Tinea versicolor
Especially on the backs of the elbows, hands, or knees or around the eyes, mouth, genitalia, or rectum	Vitiligo
Pallor in the face, nails, and inside the lower eyelids	Anemia
DARK	
Patches of hyperpigmentation, often tawny colored, especially on the chest, upper back, and neck	Tinea versicolor
Darkened face, nipples, areolae, vulva, and linea alba	Pregnancy
Darkened skin	Addison's disease
Grayish tan or bronze skin	Hemochromatosis

Erythema (redness)

ASSESSMENT FINDING	WHAT IT CAN MEAN
Red face	Alcohol intake
	Hypertension
	Fever
	Embarrassment
Localized redness	Inflammation
Petechiae and bruising	Bleeding disorder
	Vitamin C deficiency
	Medications such as warfarin
	Physical abuse
	In the elderly, may occur because of thinner, more fragile skin
Redness over pressure points	Stage I pressure ulcer

Cyanosis (bluish cast)

ASSESSMENT FINDING	WHAT IT CAN MEAN
Blue tinge to lips and tongue (central cyanosis)	Heart or lung disease
Blue tinge to nails, fingers, and toes (peripheral cyanosis)	Heart or lung disease (May accompany shock)
Reddish-blue discoloration of face, conjunctiva, mouth, hands, or feet	Polycythemia

NOTE: Lips and mucous membranes of many African-Americans normally have a red or bluish hue; patients of Mediterranean descent may have bluish lips.

Jaundice (yellowish cast)

ASSESSMENT FINDING	WHAT IT CAN MEAN
Jaundiced skin, sclera, lips, and palate	Liver or biliary tract disease
Subtle pale yellowish hue or "frost" to the skin	Chronic renal disease

ASSESSING MOISTURE, TEXTURE, AND TEMPERATURE

What you'll look for: *Oily, dry, thick, or flaky skin*

ASSESSMENT FINDING	WHAT IT CAN MEAN
Dryness	Excessive bathing Soap irritation Hypothyroidism Psoriasis
Rough, thick-textured skin	Atopic dermatitis
Very smooth, shiny skin on the legs, accompanied by brownish pigmentation	Peripheral vascular disease

Cool or warm skin

Assess temperature by using the backs of your hands.

ASSESSMENT FINDING	WHAT IT CAN MEAN
Cool	Impaired circulation Hypothyroidism
Warm	Hyperthyroidism Generalized fever Localized cellulitis Gout

Increased or decreased turgor

Check the tenderness, firmness, and depth of surface lesions by lightly palpating the skin. To assess skin turgor, lift a fold of skin on the forearm and see how it falls back into place.

ASSESSMENT FINDING	WHAT IT CAN MEAN
Taut shiny skin	Edema Scleroderma
Decreased turgor	Dehydration Malnutrition

Infestations on the scalp and in pubic hair

Check for parasites such as lice and scabies.

Loss of hair on any body part

ASSESSMENT FINDING	WHAT IT CAN MEAN
Alopecia	Tinea capitis Trichotillomania Syphilis

Nail clubbing

ASSESSMENT FINDING	WHAT IT CAN MEAN
Greater than 160° angle between fingernail and nail base	Systemic disease such a congenital cyanotic heart disease, lung cancer, and COPD

Discolored nails

ASSESSMENT FINDING	WHAT IT CAN MEAN
Lower half of nail bed is white; top half is pink or red	Chronic renal disease
Nail bed whitish to within 1 cm of tip	Cirrhosis Hypoalbuminemia

Irregular shaped nails

ASSESSMENT FINDING	WHAT IT CAN MEAN
Concave or spoon-shaped nails	Iron-deficiency anemia

ASSESSING LESIONS

Your findings may include a simple blister or a sexually transmitted disease like syphilis or herpes. Your most critical objective, however, is to look for lesions suspicious for skin cancer, especially in places where the patient can't see, such as the back, buttocks, scalp, and bottoms of the feet. Measure any suspicious lesions and refer the patient to a dermatologist or for a biopsy.

MNEMONIC FOR ASSESSING GROWTHS (YES TO ANY SUGGESTS MALIGNANCY):

A	Is the mole **A**symmetrical? Does one half look different from the other?
B	Are the **B**orders irregular?
C	Is the **C**olor uneven or irregular? Does the mole contain shades of red, white, blue, gray, or black?
D	Has the mole's **D**iameter changed recently? Is it bigger than a pencil eraser (6 mm)?
E	Has its surface area become **E**levated?

Basal cell carcinoma
(GROWS SLOWLY AND RARELY METASTASIZES)

WHEN TO SUSPECT:

- Sore has not healed for a month or more.
- Basal cell carcinoma is more common on sun-exposed areas, in men, and in fair-skinned persons over age 40.

WHAT IT LOOKS LIKE:

Pearly, semitranslucent, or waxy papule with a sharply demarcated border. Blood vessels may cover the surface and a nonhealing ulcer sometimes appears at the center. See Figure 3-1 on page 29.

Squamous cell carcinoma
(TUMOR GROWS MORE RAPIDLY THAN BASAL CELL, AND CAN METASTASIZE)

WHEN TO SUSPECT:

- Sore has not healed for a month or more.
- Squamous cell carcinoma is more common on sun-exposed areas and in fair-skinned persons over age 55.
- Actinic keratoses can develop into this cancer.

WHAT IT LOOKS LIKE:

A small, hard, cone-shaped nodule or a rough, irregular, elevated lesion. See Figure 3-2 at right.

Melanoma
(OFTEN METASTASIZES)

WHEN TO SUSPECT:

- Mole changes color or size.
- Mole bleeds, itches, or becomes painful.
- A new mole erupts.
- Melanoma is more common on a man's back and a woman's lower legs.
- Usually occurs in adults between the ages of 30 and 50.

WHAT IT LOOKS LIKE:

May have an uneven surface, irregular border, and varying pigmentation. See Figure 3-3 at right.

INTEGUMENTARY SYSTEM

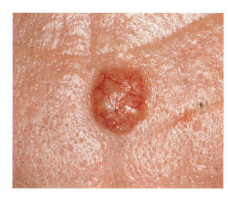

FIGURE 3-1. BASAL CELL CARCINOMAS USUALLY HAVE A WAXY, SEMI-TRANSLUCENT APPEARANCE AND A SHARPLY DEFINED BORDER.

FIGURE 3-2. SQUAMOUS CELL CARCINOMAS MAY APPEAR AS ROUGH, IRREGULAR, ELEVATED LESIONS.

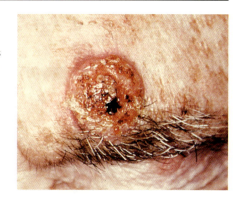

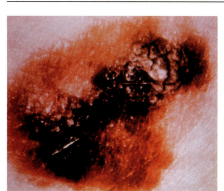

FIGURE 3-3. MALIGNANT MELANOMAS MAY HAVE AN UNEVEN SURFACE, IRREGULAR OUTLINE, AND VARYING PIGMENTATION.

FIGURE 3-4. IMPETIGO PRODUCES PUSTULES THAT BURST AND BECOME CRUSTY.

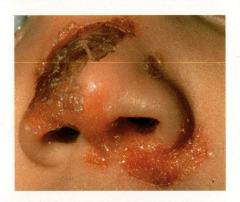

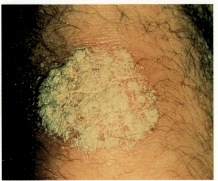

FIGURE 3-5. PSORIASIS CAUSES FLAT, CIRCUMSCRIBED LESIONS THAT OFTEN LOOK LIKE SILVERY SCALES.

FIGURE 3-6. VITILIGO, CAUSED BY AN ABSENCE OF CELLS THAT PRODUCE MELANIN, PRODUCES DEPIGMENTED PATCHES.

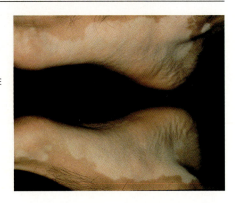

INTEGUMENTARY SYSTEM   31

FIGURE 3-7. THE SCABIES MITE BURROWS ITS WAY UNDER THE SKIN, CAUSING A SLIGHTLY ELEVATED TUNNEL.

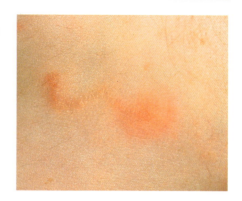

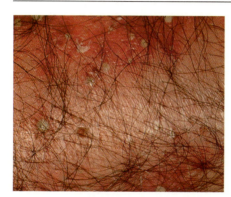

FIGURE 3-8. A STAPHYLOCOCCAL INFECTION CAN RESULT IN INFLAMED HAIR FOLLICLES AND PUSTULES.

FIGURE 3-9. A SYPHILITIC SORE, OR CHANCRE, BEGINS AS A SOLID, ELEVATED LESION AND TURNS INTO THIS REDDISH ULCER.

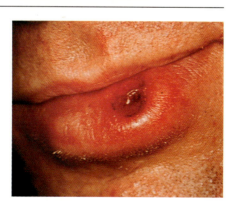

32 RN'S POCKET ASSESSMENT GUIDE

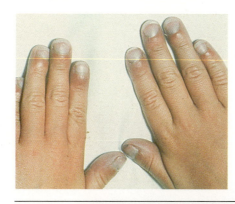

FIGURE 3-10. CLUBBING OF NAILS MAY BE A SIGN OF HEART OR LUNG DISEASE.

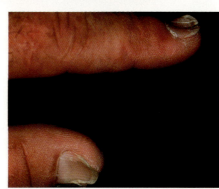

FIGURE 3-11. SPOON-SHAPED NAILS, CALLED KOILONYCHIA, MAY SIGNAL IRON-DEFICIENCY ANEMIA.

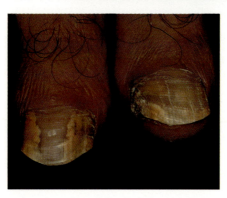

FIGURE 3-12. FUNGAL INFECTIONS IN THE NAILS, CALLED ONYCHOMYCOSIS, CAN MAKE THE NAIL PLATE THICK AND OPAQUE.

DOCUMENTING YOUR FINDINGS

- Note the location of lesions and whether they are localized, regionalized, or scattered over the entire skin surface.
- Note the size of lesions and their configuration:
  Straight line?
  Arc-shaped (arciform)?
  Round (annular)?
  Dermatomal
  (follows a nerve on one side of the body,
  as with herpes zoster)?
- Note skin findings for mucous membranes, hair, and scalp.
- Note the appearance of lesions (e.g., color) and any accompanying symptoms such as tenderness.

CHAPTER FOUR

Head, neck, and cranial nerves

The "head" part of your head-to-toe assessment will help you uncover impairments in areas basic to human function and interaction: Seeing. Hearing. Smelling. Talking. Swallowing.

A neurological exam starts with a check of level of consciousness and moves on to an evaluation of the 12 pairs of cranial nerves. Knowing the functions of these nerves and how to test them will help you detect sensory and motor deficits resulting from neurological disorders such as head trauma, stroke, brain tumor, or meningitis. Dysfunction can also occur following neurosurgery or surgery of the face or neck.

SYSTEM REVIEW SHOULD COVER:

HEAD:

- Dizziness
- Headaches
- Pain
- Fainting
- History of head injury
- Loss of consciousness
- Stroke
- Limitation of movement (range of motion)

EYES:

- Use of eyeglasses, contact lenses, or prosthetics
- Current vision
- Change in vision
- Double vision (diplopia)
- Excess tearing
- Pain
- Recent eye examinations
- Pain when looking at light (photophobia)
- Unusual sensations
- Redness
- Discharge
- Infections
- History of glaucoma
- Cataracts
- Injuries
- Medications
- Eye surgery

EARS:

- Hearing impairment
- Use of hearing aids
- Discharge
- Pain
- Ringing in ears
- Infections
- History of ear trauma

NOSE:

- Nosebleeds
- Infections
- Discharge
- Frequency of colds
- Nasal obstruction
- History of injury
- Sinus infections
- Hay fever
- Nasal surgery
- Use of nasal medications

MOUTH AND THROAT:

- Bleeding gums
- Frequent sore throats
- Burning of tongue
- Dental care

NECK:

- Lumps
- Goiter
- Pain on movement
- Tenderness
- History of swollen glands
- Thyroid trouble

LEVEL OF CONSCIOUSNESS (LOC)

ASSESSING LOC:

Is the patient awake?

If yes, is he oriented to person, place, and time?
(For a discussion on assessing mental status in conscious patients, see Chapter 5, Nervous System.)

If no, does he awaken when you call his name?

If no, does he respond to shouting?

If no, does he respond to gentle shaking?

If no, does he respond to pain? Compress the supraorbital area with your thumbs. If the patient has a facial injury, apply pressure to the nail beds or squeeze the Achilles tendon instead. Test both sides of the body.

If he responds to pain, how does he respond
(e.g., does he pull away from the stimulus or grimace)?

Is there decorticate posturing (abnormal flexion)?
This indicates a disruption of the corticospinal pathways.

Is there decerebrate posturing (abnormal extension)?
This indicates damage closer to the brain stem, in the area of the midbrain or pons.

DOCUMENTING LOC:

When describing level of consciousness, avoid such unspecific terms as lethargic, stuporous, or obtunded. Instead, report the stimulus you used, the duration you used it, and the response to it. For example: "Opens eyes briefly when name is called," or "No response after 30 seconds of pressure to the nail beds."

Use a standard assessment tool such as the Glasgow Coma Scale (GCS) below to document your finding. Rate your patient according to his best response to stimuli. Someone who's alert and oriented will have a perfect score of 15; a deeply comatose patient might score only 3.

GLASGOW COMA SCALE

EYES OPEN	Spontaneously	4
Record C	To speech	3
if eyes closed	To pain	2
by swelling	No response	1
BEST MOTOR	Obeys commands	6
RESPONSE	Localizes pain	5
Record best	Flexion-withdrawal	4
upper arm response	Abnormal flexion	3
	Abnormal extension	2
	No response	1
BEST VERBAL	Oriented	5
RESPONSE	Confused	4
Record T if	Inappropriate words	3
endotracheal	Incomprehensible	2
or tracheostomy	sounds	
tube in place	No response	1

TOTAL SCORE

FIGURE 4-1. ABNORMAL FLEXION.

The arms hyperflex while the legs hyperextend and rotate inward.

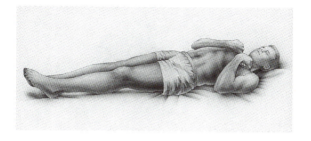

FIGURE 4-2. ABNORMAL EXTENSION.

The arms and legs hyperextend and there is hyperpronation of the arms.

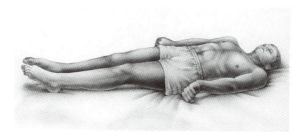

40 RN'S POCKET ASSESSMENT GUIDE

FIGURE 4-3. A QUICK LOOK AT CRANIAL NERVE FUNCTION

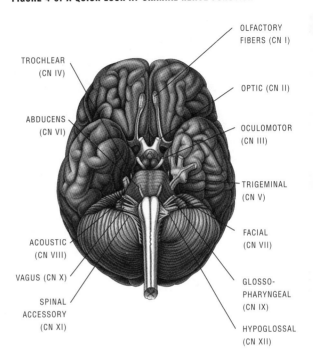

CRANIAL NERVE	TYPE	FUNCTION
I Olfactory	Sensory	Smell
II Optic	Sensory	Visual acuity, field of vision, pupillary response (afferent impulse)
III Oculomotor	Motor	Eyelid elevation, extraocular movement, pupil size, convergence, pupillary constriction (efferent impulse)
IV Trochlear	Motor	Extraocular movement
V Trigeminal	Sensory, motor	Facial sensation, corneal reflex, chewing
VI Abducens	Motor	Extraocular movement
VII Facial	Sensory, motor	Taste, corneal reflex, facial expression
VIII Acoustic	Sensory	Hearing, equilibrium
IX Glossopharyngeal	Sensory, motor	Taste, gagging, swallowing
X Vagus	Sensory, motor	Speech (vocal quality), gagging, swallowing
XI Spinal accessory	Motor	Head rotation, shoulder movement
XII Hypoglossal	Motor	Tongue movement, speech (articulation)

ASSESSING CRANIAL NERVES

Whether you are testing sensory or motor function, be certain to assess the face and body bilaterally. Test each nerve or group of nerves in numerical order. This way you'll learn to associate each nerve with its function without missing any.

What you'll need:

- Aromatic substance such as coffee
- Snellen chart
- Newspaper or other reading matter
- Red pen or other brightly colored object
- Penlight
- Cotton
- Tongue blade
- Tuning fork
- Cotton-tipped applicator

Olfactory nerve (CN I)

TEST SMELL
(Test only if the patient has a head injury or reports an impaired or absent sense of smell.)

Have the patient close his eyes and occlude one nostril. Under the other one, hold something with a familiar aroma, such as coffee. See if he can identify it.

NOTE: Don't use pungent, irritating substances such as ammonia or alcohol. They stimulate the pain fibers carried by the trigeminal nerve and will interfere with the response you want to elicit. Keep in mind that cigarette smoking, cocaine use, inflammation, rhinitis, or sinus problems can all interfere with the sense of smell.

Absence of smell—anosmia—related to cranial nerve dysfunction is most often the result of a head injury, particularly a basilar skull fracture, or a tumor of the olfactory groove. Other causes include a vitamin B_{12} deficiency and advanced syphilis.

Optic nerve (CN II)

TEST GROSS VISION	Use a Snellen chart or, if you don't have one, a newspaper. Hold it 20 feet from the patient. With his glasses or contacts in place, have him cover one eye and read the headlines. If he can't do that, hold up several fingers and ask him to count them.
TEST NEAR VISION	Hand the patient the newspaper—or a menu or education brochure—and ask him to read it. Test each eye separately. If the patient is unable to read, show pictures and see if he can identify them.
TEST VISUAL FIELDS	Use the confrontation technique: Stand facing the patient, an arm's length away. Have him cover his right eye while you cover your left. Ask him to look at your uncovered eye. Hold a brightly colored object, such as a red pen, in your other hand and extend that arm out to the side.

Slowly move the object from the periphery to the center of the visual field—the midpoint between your eye and the patient's. Have the patient say "now" when he first sees the object. You both should notice it at the same time.

Repeat the test several times for each eye, moving the pen in from a different direction each time, as shown in Figure 4-4. If the patient is confused or uncooperative, use the startle technique: Moving the pen with a flickering motion, observe for a blink response.

Be alert for scotomas—areas of decreased or absent vision. If the patient has suffered a stroke, you may detect hemianopsia— depressed vision or blindness in half of the visual field.

FIGURE 4-4. TESTING VISUAL FIELDS WITH THE CONFRONTATION TECHNIQUE.

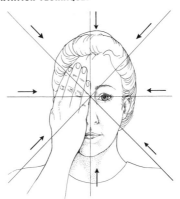

Oculomotor nerve (CN III)

ASSESS PUPILS

Note size, shape, and symmetry. Normal pupils are round and equal in size, ranging from 3–7 mm in diameter, although anisocoria—inequality in size—can be congenital.

TEST RESPONSE TO LIGHT
(a function of both CN II and CN III)

The lights in the room should be dim. If the patient is conscious, have him look straight ahead and focus on something in the distance. Hold a penlight in his peripheral field of vision, and shine it obliquely—not directly—on the pupil. Both the target pupil—the one receiving the light—and the opposite pupil should constrict briskly. (Constriction of the target pupil is known as the direct response; of the opposite pupil, the consensual response. If a patient is blind in one eye and you shine a light in that eye, neither pupil will react. But if you shine the light in the opposite eye, both pupils should constrict.)

NOTE: Certain drugs and ophthalmic medications cause pupils to dilate or constrict. In addition, cataracts can interfere with the pupils' ability to respond to light. A sluggish pupillary response when none of these factors are involved can indicate increased intracranial pressure.

TEST ACCOMMODATION
(the ability of eyes to adjust to objects at various distances)

Hold your finger about 12 inches in front of the patient while he focuses on some distant point. Then ask him to look at your finger. As he switches focus, the pupils should constrict. The eyes should also converge, or cross.

FIGURE 4-5. WHICH NERVES CONTROL EYE MOVEMENT.

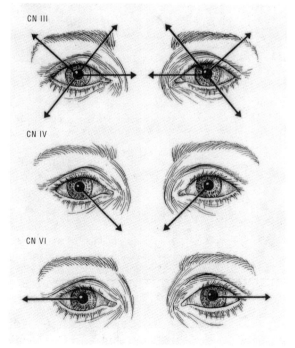

Extraocular nerves
(CN III, CN IV, CN VI)

TEST EYE MOVEMENT

Ask the patient to look up, down, laterally, and diagonally. Or have him track your finger as you draw the letter H in the air about 18 inches in front of him. The patient should be able to move his eyes in all directions.

While assessing extraocular movements (EOM), look for nystagmus—rapid involuntary movements of the eyeballs. A few beats of nystagmus on prolonged lateral gaze may be normal.

ASSESS EYELID ELEVATION
(CN III)

With eyes open, the lid should cover no more than one-third of the iris. A patient who has a CN III lesion may have ptosis—drooping of the eyelid. Since this nerve controls the upward, downward, diagonal, and medial movements of the eye as well, the patient may only be able to move his eye laterally.

Trigeminal nerve (CN V)

TEST FACIAL SENSATION

Ask the patient to close his eyes. Brush his forehead, cheeks, and chin with a piece of cotton. Have him say "now" when he feels the stimulus.

If the patient is unconscious, test the corneal reflex instead. Touch the cornea lightly with a wisp of sterile cotton. The normal response is bilateral blinking.

TEST MOTOR FUNCTION OF TEMPORAL AND MASSETER MUSCLES

Ask the patient to clench his teeth while you palpate his temples and jaw. Movement should be symmetrical, and the jaw shouldn't deviate.

Test muscle strength by having him bite down on a tongue blade with his back teeth. Ask him to move his jaw laterally against resistance. Then place your hand beneath his chin, and instruct him to open his mouth while you try to hold it shut.

Facial nerve (CN VII)

TEST MOTOR FUNCTION

Observe the face at rest. Look for such signs of weakness as a drooping mouth or asymmetrical nasolabial folds. Then ask the patient to smile, frown, close his eyes, raise his eyebrows, wrinkle his forehead, show his teeth, puff out his cheeks, and say "me me me" or purse his lips and whistle.

HEAD, NECK, AND CRANIAL NERVES **49**

	To test muscle strength against resistance, see if he can keep his eyes closed as you gently try to pry them open.
TEST TASTE *(not routinely tested)*	Have the patient stick out his tongue. Place some salt or sugar on the sides and see if he can identify it.

Acoustic nerve (CN VIII)

TEST GROSS HEARING	Have the patient cover one ear. Hold a ticking watch or run your fingers together a few inches from his other ear. Or stand about two feet behind him and whisper a two-digit number. Repeat with other ear.
	If you suspect hearing loss in one ear, do the Weber test: Strike a tuning fork and place it on top of the patient's head, centering it. If he has a conductive hearing loss—caused by a defect in the middle or outer ear—the sound will be louder in the affected ear. If the problem is sensorineural—caused by inner ear or acoustic nerve damage—he'll hear it better in the unaffected ear.
CHECK EQUILIBRIUM	Ask the patient if he experiences dizziness, vertigo, or loss of balance.

Glossopharyngeal nerve (CN IX) and vagus nerve (CN X)

TEST GAG AND SWALLOWING REFLEXES	With the patient sitting upright, have him open his mouth. Depress the tongue with a tongue blade and touch the throat with a cotton-tipped applicator. As the pharyngeal muscles contract, the patient should gag. If the vagus nerve is intact, he'll also be able to feel the blade.
	Next have the patient say "ah" while you look in his mouth. The uvula should rise but not deviate to either side. Ask the patient to swallow. If CN IX and CN X are both intact, he should be able to do so without difficulty.
ASSESS SPEECH *(partly controlled by CN X)*	Listen to the patient talk; if his voice sounds nasal, he may have pharyngeal paralysis. Then ask him to make a squeaking sound. Hoarseness or an inability to make high-pitched sounds can signal vocal cord weakness.

Spinal accessory nerve (CN XI)

TEST STERNOCLEIDOMASTOID MUSCLE STRENGTH	Have the patient turn his head while you hold your hand against his cheek.
TEST TRAPEZIUS MUSCLE STRENGTH	Ask him to shrug his shoulders while you press down on them.

Hypoglossal nerve (CN XII)

ASSESS FOR MILD DYSARTHRIA	See if the patient has difficulty saying "la la la" or a word or phrase with consonants, such as "Massachusetts." Observe his tongue at rest, then ask him to stick it out. With a lesion of CN XII, the tongue deviates to the weak side.
TEST LINGUAL STRENGTH	Have the patient move his tongue from side to side, then try to lift it while you press down with a tongue blade. Or have him push his tongue against the inside of the cheek while you press his cheek from the outside.

Disorders affecting specific cranial nerves

While neurological conditions such as stroke, head trauma, and increased intracranial pressure may involve several nerves, certain disorders are related to just one. Some of the more common are listed below.

DISORDER	CRANIAL NERVE	SIGNS AND SYMPTOMS	POSSIBLE CAUSES
TRIGEMINAL NEURALGIA (*tic douloureux*)	V	Recurrent attacks of tics and intense shooting or burning pain in one side of the face; pain may be triggered by light touch, cold, or pressure to sensitive areas.	Irritation or compression of the nerve by a blood vessel Trauma to or infection of the teeth or jaw Viral illness, e.g., herpes zoster Multiple sclerosis Brain tumor or infarction
BELL'S PALSY (*facial paralysis*)	VII	Facial or periauricular discomfort or pain, progressing to one-sided facial paralysis. Inability to smile, whistle, grimace, or close the eye. Diminished taste.	Swelling of the nerve due to vasculitis or viral or immune disease, resulting in nerve compression, ischemia, and degeneration Local ischemia, edema, or infarction Intracranial tumor or hemorrhage

MENIERE'S DISEASE	VIII	Recurrent attacks of vertigo, which may be accompanied by tinnitus, nystagmus, hearing loss, nausea, vomiting, and a feeling of pressure or fullness in the ear; hearing loss may progress to deafness.	Excess fluid accumulation in the ear's membranous labyrinth, leading to cochlear degeneration Allergy Toxicity Local ischemia Hypoxia or hemorrhage
GLOSSOPHARYNGEAL NEURALGIA	IX	Pain in the throat and, in some cases, the ear, which may be triggered by chewing, swallowing, laughing, yawning, or blowing the nose.	Nerve inflammation, compression, or injury Herpes zoster

CHAPTER FIVE

Nervous system

You may not think about it, but you perform some type of neurological assessment every day—simply by observing how a patient feeds himself, gets out of bed, or carries out other activities of daily living. Indeed, the simple art of shaking hands reveals a great deal of information. During history-taking, you can learn about mental status, gait, stance, motor power, and coordination.

There will be times, however, when a patient needs a more complete assessment: upon admission, after trauma or cranial surgery, for example, or when a neurological disorder is suspected. Adding the following techniques to your repertoire of assessment skills will help you identify your patient's strengths and weaknesses and determine the extent of any neurological deficits.

SYSTEM REVIEW SHOULD COVER:

- Weakness
- Paralysis
- Muscle stiffness
- Limitation of movement (range of motion)
- Fainting
- Dizziness
- Blackouts
- Strokes
- Numbness
- Tingling (paresthesia)
- Burning
- Tremors
- Loss of memory
- Psychiatric disorders
- Mood changes
- Nervousness
- Speech disorders
- Unsteadiness of gait
- General behavioral change
- Hallucinations
- Disorientation, confusion

SPECIFIC QUESTIONS TO ASK:

- What is your name? Where are you now? What is today's date? What year is it?
- Do you know why you have come to the hospital?
- Do you have any other medical problems?
- Have you had any dizziness, headaches, blackouts, neck stiffness, blurred vision, loss of memory, or speech and swallowing difficulties?
- Have you been experiencing nausea, vomiting, numbness, tingling, weakness, or clumsiness?
- Do you lose your balance or fall?
- Do you have difficulty urinating?
- Are you incontinent?
- Do you take any prescription or over-the-counter medications?
- Do you drink alcohol or use any illicit drugs? If so, how often?
- Have you been exposed to toxic agents?
- Does your family have any history of cardiovascular disease or hereditary neurological disorders, such as Huntington's chorea and neurofibromatosis?

ASSESSING MENTAL STATUS

- Note whether the patient responds readily and appropriately to questions. Difficulty understanding questions could be a sign of receptive aphasia; difficulty choosing the right words to answer could be a sign of expressive aphasia.

- If you suspect expressive aphasia, test for it by showing the patient a few simple objects, such as a pen, pad, and thermometer, and asking him to name them. Listen for hoarseness, nasal speech, or slurring of words—any of which may indicate muscle or nerve damage.

- If the patient understands simple questions, see whether both sides of his brain are working together by having him follow a three-step command (e.g., tell him to pick up a cup of water in his left hand, take a sip, then put the cup down using his right hand).

- Note past memory with questions about prior hospitalizations. Check recent memory by asking the patient what he had for breakfast. Or, recite three or four unrelated words and have him repeat them. Five minutes later, ask him to say them again.

- To assess affect, ask the patient to describe how he's feeling and watch his facial expression. Does it match the emotions he's describing? Does he appear anxious or depressed?

- Note the patient's attention span. Is he easily distracted?

- To assess judgment, note whether the patient is dressed appropriately for the weather and the occasion (though it's possible he has only one set of clothes). You can also present him with a cause and effect situation: What would he do if he smelled smoke in a crowded room?

- To assess ability to reason abstractly, have the patient interpret a proverb such as "Don't put all your eggs in one basket," or perform a simple calculation. Take into account his educational level and cultural background when framing your questions. Knowledge should be appropriate to the patient's age, education, occupation, and cultural background.

ASSESSING MUSCLE TONE AND STRENGTH

This part of the neuro exam will help you detect disorders of the motor cortex, the descending motor tracts, the spinal cord, and the peripheral nerves. Visually divide the body in half, and check for symmetry of shape, size, and strength—the hallmarks of an intact neuromuscular system. Focus on the trunk and the extremities. When checking motor function, observe the muscles first at rest and then in action.

General inspection

With the patient seated in a chair or sitting or lying in bed, ask him to take several deep breaths to relax his muscles. Look for atrophy, contractures, asymmetry, and any involuntary movements—tics, twitches, jerks, or tremors.

Muscle tone

Passively flex and extend each limb. There should be slight resistance upon flexion and extension.

Spasticity (increased tone upon first stretching the muscle) can occur, for example, with spinal cord injury, after spinal shock has resolved, and after stroke.

Rigidity (increased tone that persists throughout the range of motion exercise) is seen in Parkinson's disease and other disorders of the extrapyramidal system. It's often accompanied by tremors and tends to decrease with voluntary movement.

Flaccidity (absence of muscle tone) can occur with a number of conditions, including spinal shock or stroke. A flaccid limb will feel heavy and limp as you move it, and will fall abruptly if you lift and then release it.

Muscle strength

UPPER EXTREMITIES	Ask the patient to try to extend his arm while you hold it in a flexed position. Then have him attempt to flex it while you hold it in extension.
GRIP	Have the patient squeeze your first two fingers.
PROXIMAL ARM	Have the patient close his eyes and hold his arms out in front of him for at least 15 seconds, with palms facing up.

A weak arm will drift downward, and the thumb will rotate inward. A slight drift (pronator drift) can indicate pressure on the motor cortex, caused by a brain tumor, head injury, or stroke. |
| **LEGS** | Place a hand on the patient's thigh and ask him to lift his leg while you press down. Then remove your hand and |

	have him raise each leg, without bending the knee, as high as he can. Pain during this maneuver can signal a lower back problem.
THIGHS	Have him flex his feet at the ankles—dorsiflexion—and press his toes against your hand—plantar flexion. Make sure he can wiggle his toes.
	Unless he's on bed rest or is hemodynamically unstable, ask him to sit on the edge of the bed and then stand up, without using his arms.

HOW TO GRADE THE STRENGTH OF ARM AND LEG MUSCLES:

0	No muscle contraction
1	Flicker or trace of contraction
2	Active movement with gravity eliminated—patient can move limb from side to side
3	Active movement against gravity—patient can lift limb
4	Active movement against gravity and moderate resistance
5	Full range of motion against gravity and resistance (normal strength)

ASSESSING BALANCE AND COORDINATION

SPINE	With the patient standing and bending forward, assess for deformities such as scoliosis.
GAIT	As the patient walks, assess muscle strength, coordination, and balance.

Mild gait problems can occur in the elderly, but a young or middle-aged adult should not exhibit unsteadiness, loss of balance, a widened stance, dragging of one foot, shuffling, or staggering.

If the patient's gait is normal, ask him to walk on tiptoe to test the strength of his calf muscles. Then have him walk on his heels. Someone with peroneal nerve damage won't be able to do the test.

ROMBERG TEST

To test balance, ask him to close his eyes and remain still, with his feet together. Stand close to the patient so you can steady him if he starts to fall. (If he's unsteady even with his eyes open, don't perform the Romberg test.)

The patient may sway slightly, but he shouldn't fall or break his stance. If he does, it could signal peripheral neuropathy or spinal cord damage.

WALKING

Have the patient walk in a straight line, heel to toe, and check his balance.

If the patient is confined to bed, assess for cerebellar ataxia—lack of muscle coordination—by having him run the heel of one foot down the shin of the other leg.

COORDINATION AND POSITION SENSE	Hold your forefinger an arm's length from the patient. Have him repeatedly touch his forefinger to yours and then to his nose, alternating as rapidly as possible. Then, move your target finger to the left or right, and have him perform the exercise again.
FINE MOTOR COORDINATION	Ask the patient to tap his thumb with each of the fingers on the same hand in succession.

ASSESSING REFLEXES

What you'll need:

■ Reflex hammer

FIGURE 5-1. TESTING THE BICEPS REFLEX.

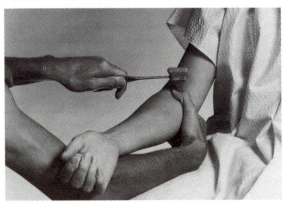

Have the patient flex his arm slightly, palm up. Hold his arm at the elbow, with your thumb over the biceps tendon in the antecubital space. Strike your thumb with the reflex hammer. The biceps muscle should contract and the arm should flex slightly.

NERVOUS SYSTEM **63**

FIGURE 5-2. TESTING THE TRICEPS TENDON.

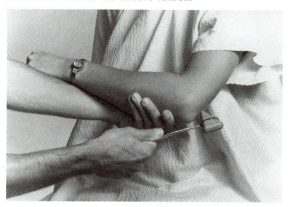

Have the patient flex his arm at a 90° angle. With his arm supported by your hand, strike the triceps tendon between the epicondyles just above the elbow. The tendon should contract, the elbow extend.

FIGURE 5-3. TESTING THE BRACHIORADIALIS REFLEX.

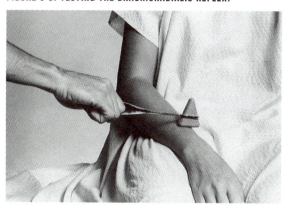

Have the patient rest his arm—flexed slightly with palm face down—on his lap. Strike the radius about two inches above the wrist. The forearm should rotate laterally and the palm turn upward.

FIGURE 5-4. TESTING THE PATELLAR REFLEX.

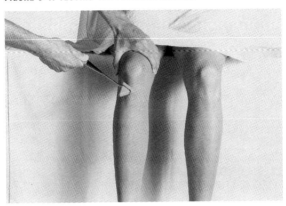

Have the patient dangle his legs over the side of the bed.
Place your hand on the patient's thigh, and strike the distal patellar tendon just below the kneecap. The quadriceps muscle should contract, the knee extend.

FIGURE 5-5. TESTING THE ACHILLES TENDON REFLEX.

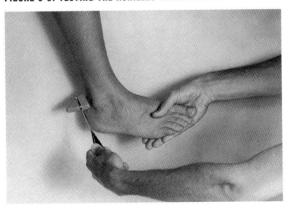

Have the patient dorsiflex his foot slightly. Lightly strike the Achilles tendon. The foot should plantar flex.

NERVOUS SYSTEM

ASSESSMENT FINDING	WHAT IT CAN MEAN
Hyperactive reflexes	Upper motor neuron disease Electrolyte imbalance Preeclampsia
Diminished or absent reflexes (areflexia)	Lower motor neuron disease Electrolyte imbalance

HOW TO GRADE REFLEX ACTIVITY:

0	No reflex
1	Sluggish
2	Normal
3	Brisk
4	Hyperactive

In addition to assessing deep tendon reflexes, check for Babinski's sign—upward movement of the big toe, with fanning of the other toes. The presence of Babinski's sign may indicate upper motor neuron or corticospinal disease.

FIGURE 5-6. CHECKING FOR BABINSKI'S SIGN.
Stroke the sole of the foot with a semi-sharp object, such as the handle of a reflex hammer, as shown here. (In ticklish patients, stroke the area beneath the external malleolus.) In adults and children older than 2, the toes normally flex downward.

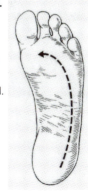

ASSESSING SENSATION

What you'll need:

- Cotton ball and swab
- Suitable sharp object
- Specimen tubes
- Tuning fork

SUPERFICIAL PAIN SENSATION	First, brush a cotton ball against the skin of the patient's arms and legs to find out if he can feel a light touch. Then, using a suitable sharp object (e.g., a wooden cotton-tipped applicator or tongue blade broken in half), touch the patient once or twice in each foot, lower leg, thigh, hand, forearm, and upper arm. Touch with the sharp end—taking care not to penetrate the skin—then with the dull or soft end. Ask the patient to tell you whether the sensation feels sharp or dull.
TEMPERATURE SENSATION *(Test if response to pain is diminished.)*	Apply specimen tubes with hot and cold water to the area of diminished response, and have the patient tell you what he feels.
RESPONSE TO VIBRATION	Use a C-128 tuning fork. Strike the fork, apply it to a bony prominence on the back of his hand, and count seconds. Have the patient report when the vibrations stop. A normal response lasts 15 to 20 seconds, though sensation may be diminished in the elderly.

If the response is abnormal, repeat the test on the wrist, and compare the patient's reaction with your own. Move the fork up the arm along the bony prominences until findings are in the normal range.

To test the lower extremities, start with the toes. If the patient can't feel the vibrations, try the ankle, then the tibia. A normal response over the tibia lasts about 10 seconds.

Again, move up the leg until sensation is normal.

PROPRIOCEPTION

With the patient's eyes closed, grasp the sides of one toe's distal joint and move it slightly up or down, being careful not to touch the adjacent digits. Ask the patient to tell you which way you're moving it; he should be able to feel even the slightest movement.

Repeat exercise at least three times with different toes, and document the number of correct responses.

Repeat exercise using the fingers.

FINE SENSATION

Snap a cotton swab in half, and use the soft tips to touch two areas of the skin simultaneously. The patient should be able to distinguish between two points less than 4 mm apart on the fingertips—the most sensitive area.

STEREOGNOSIS	Place a small object such as a paper clip in the patient's hand and ask him to identify it. Test each hand separately and don't allow him to pass the object from hand to hand.
GRAPHESTHESIA	Trace a number on the patient's palm and ask him to identify it.

CHAPTER SIX

Respiratory system

Taking a thorough patient history and skillfully using a stethoscope are your top priorities when assessing the pulmonary tree. If the patient is in respiratory distress, however, keep your history brief. Ask as many Yes or No questions—ones that can be answered by a nod or shake of the head—as possible, or obtain information from medical records or family members. Then do a quick inspection and move directly to the auscultation segment of your physical exam.

SYSTEM REVIEW SHOULD COVER:

- Cough
- Pain
- Shortness of breath
- Sputum production (quantity, appearance)
- Tuberculosis
- Asthma
- COPD
- Coughing up blood (hemoptysis)
- Wheezing
- Last chest X-ray
- Last test for tuberculosis
- History of TB vaccination

SPECIFIC QUESTIONS TO ASK:

- Do you need to prop yourself up on several pillows at night to breath comfortably (orthopnea)?
- Has there been a recent change in the amount, color, or consistency of mucus?
- Do you have exercise-induced asthma?
- Do you have allergies?
- How would you rate any present respiratory distress on a scale of 0 to 10? How do present symptoms compare with those of previous attacks?
- Have you been given any skin tests for allergies or fungal infections? If so, what were the results?
- Do you take any prescription or over-the-counter medications?
- Have you received vaccines to prevent pneumonia, influenza, and tetanus?
- Have you had a skin test for tuberculosis?
- When did you last have a chest X-ray?
- Have you experienced any chest trauma or had any surgery that involved the chest?
- Do you now, or have you ever, smoked? If so, how many cigarettes a day and for how many years?

- Are you exposed to secondary smoke, asbestos, coal dust, fumes from paint, airplane glue, or furniture refinishing products—or potentially toxic particles from other sources—either at work or at home?
- How well ventilated is the site? Is your home near a factory or source of air pollution?
- Have you traveled recently? If so, where?
- Does any family member suffer from an infectious or genetic disorder that affects the respiratory system, including tuberculosis, pneumonia, bronchitis, or cystic fibrosis?
- Do you have alpha$_1$-antitrypsin deficiency (an inherited condition that leads to emphysema)?

ASSESSING SHAPE, SYMMETRY, AND SKIN

Once your history is complete, proceed with the physical exam. The patient should be seated, with his chest exposed. Note whether the patient has to sit straight up or lean forward to breathe comfortably. If the patient can't sit up by himself, get assistance, or roll him onto his side.

Since many respiratory abnormalities are unilateral or localized, compare findings on one side of the body with those on the other. Also compare front with back. Record your findings with reference to the standard lines illustrated in Figure 6-1 on page 74.

What you'll need:

- Tape measure

What you'll inspect:

Shape and symmetry of the chest and spine

What you should find:

- The anterior-posterior diameter of the chest is approximately one-third to one-half the side-to-side diameter.
- The vertebral line is straight.

ABNORMAL FINDING	SIGNIFICANCE
BARREL CHEST Increased anterior-posterior diameter	May signal air trapping, the result of conditions such as pneumothorax, asthma, and emphysema. In the elderly, barrel chest may be the result of loss of elasticity of the lungs.
FUNNEL CHEST (PECTUS EXCAVATUM) Depression of the sternum	Congenital condition; patients are usually asymptomatic. If severe, though, can cause respiratory failure.
PIGEON CHEST (PECTUS CARINATUM) Forward protrusion of the sternum, either at the xiphoid process or center of the sternum	Patients with the congenital form are usually asymptomatic. Those with acquired pigeon chest, which often results from atrial or ventricular defects, may be at risk for pulmonary hypertension.
SCOLIOSIS Side to side deviation of the spine's curvature	Severe scoliosis reduces chest wall compliance, causing restrictive pulmonary disease.

KYPHOSCOLIOSIS
Convex front-to-back curvature of the thoracic spine (kyphosis) and scoliosis

Can contribute to chest infection and respiratory failure by inhibiting lung expansion and the ability to cough effectively.

Chest symmetry as the patient breathes

ABNORMAL FINDING	WHAT IT CAN MEAN
Delay in chest wall movement over one side	Localized disease, including pneumothorax, atelectasis, pneumonia, rib fractures, and partial paralysis of the diaphragm, or scoliosis
Reduced chest expansion on both sides	Neuromuscular diseases or COPD
Bulging or retraction of the intercostal muscles, the sternocleidomastoid muscles of the neck, and the trapezius muscles, between the back of the neck and the shoulders	Respiratory distress

Skin color

ABNORMAL FINDING	WHAT IT CAN MEAN
Cyanosis in the lips and mucous membranes of the mouth (central cyanosis)	Low arterial saturation, resulting from inadequate gas exchange in the lungs or cardiac shunting. Occasionally accompanies COPD and other primary pulmonary disorders.

(Continued)

74 RN'S POCKET ASSESSMENT GUIDE

FIGURE 6-1. THORACIC LANDMARKS. Letters signify commonly used auscultation points for bronchial (B), bronchovesicular (BV), and vesicular (V) breath sounds.

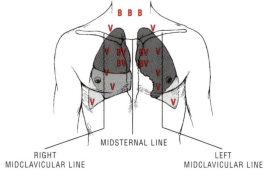
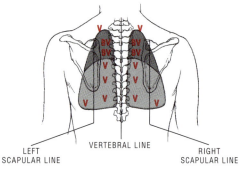
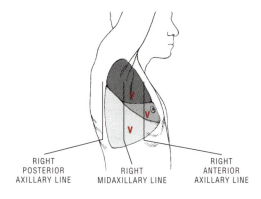

ABNORMAL FINDING	WHAT IT CAN MEAN
Cyanosis in the fingers, toes, and tip of the nose (peripheral cyanosis)	Low venous saturation, resulting from too much oxygen being extracted by the tissues. Occurs in shock and other disorders that reduce cardiac output.
Pallor	Respiratory distress, although it can result from anemia or another chronic disease.
Flushed, ruddy complexion, accompanied by fever and labored breathing	Excess CO_2 and, possibly, impending respiratory failure.

ASSESSING BREATHING

Observe the rate, rhythm, and depth of the patient's breathing for one full minute.

What you should find:

- Adults: 12–20 breaths per minute.
- Elderly: 16–25 breaths per minute.
- Exhaling takes about twice as long as inhaling (in COPD patients it may take up to four times longer).
- Rhythm is even, with occasional sighs.

ABNORMAL FINDING	WHAT IT CAN MEAN
CHEYNE-STOKES RESPIRATIONS Rhythmic increase and decrease in depth, punctuated by regular episodes of apnea	Severe heart failure Uremia Neurological disorder (In the elderly, Cheyne-Stokes respirations may be normal.)
TACHYPNEA Rapid breathing with no change in depth	Pain Anxiety Fever Anemia

(Continued)

ABNORMAL FINDING	WHAT IT CAN MEAN
HYPERPNEA **(KUSSMAUL'S RESPIRATIONS)** Rapid, deep breathing	Diabetic ketoacidosis and other forms of metabolic acidosis (Hyperpnea also occurs normally during strenuous exercise.)
HYPOPNEA Abnormal decrease in depth and rate of breathing	Change in mental status Severe hypoxia Acute drug or alcohol intoxication
DYSPNEA Difficult, labored, or painful breathing	Any disorder that interferes with pulmonary function
BIOT'S RESPIRATIONS Irregular breathing punctuated by apnea every four or five cycles	Meningitis or another neurological disorder

NOTES:
Pursed lip breathing may indicate COPD, but it is not always a sign of acute respiratory distress, since patients with long-standing disease are taught how to use this technique to make breathing easier.

Nasal flaring suggests respiratory distress, especially in children. May also signal dyspnea in patients on mechanical ventilation.

PALPATING THE CHEST WALL

Begin palpation by using the palms of both hands to assess the entire chest for tenderness, depressions, and bulges. Crepitus—a palpable crunching that feels like Rice Krispies® or cellophane under the skin—may indicate the presence of air in subcutaneous tissues. It can sometimes be elicited in a patient who's had a chest injury, pneumothorax, or tracheostomy.

FIGURE 6-2. ASSESSING CHEST WALL MOVEMENT AND SYMMETRY.

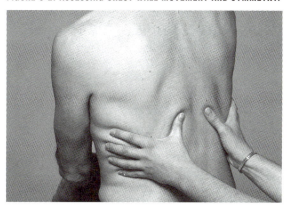

Place the hands between the eighth and 10th posterior ribs and have the patient breathe deeply. As he inhales, each hand should move about 3–5 cm from the spine.

FIGURE 6-3. DETERMINING IF THE TRACHEA HAS BEEN DISPLACED.

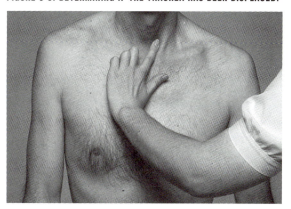

Place your index finger first on the right side of the suprasternal notch, then on the left. If lateral displacement has occurred—as a result of tension pneumothorax, for example—you'll feel the trachea on one side and soft tissue on the other.

FIGURE 6-4. EVALUATING VOCAL FREMITUS.

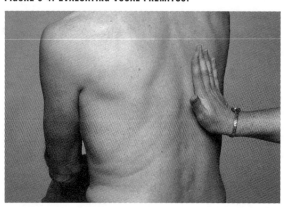

Gently place the ball of the hand in the upper back and have the patient repeat the words "ninety-nine." Evaluate the intensity of the vibration over all lung fields, comparing side to side. Diseases that increase lung density increase the intensity of vocal vibrations, while those that trap air diminish the sound.

PERCUSSING FOR GROSS DEFECTS

Sounds generated by percussion indicate density of lung tissue to a depth of 5–7 cm. Percussion isn't helpful in detecting subtle abnormalities, however. It's best to perform it over the patient's back, as the heart and breasts interfere with anterior assessment.

To cover the entire chest, percuss systematically at 3–5 cm intervals, starting just above the scapulae and moving from side to side and downward, avoiding the scapulae and spine. Document any differences in volume and pitch.

What you'll hear:

RESONANCE	Loud, long, low-pitched sound. Can generally be heard over most lung fields.
HYPERRESONANCE	A loud, very long sound, lower-pitched than resonance. May signal emphysema or tension pneumothorax, though it can be normal in very thin patients.
DULLNESS OR FLATNESS	Dullness is a medium-pitched sound of medium duration and medium intensity; flatness, a soft, high-pitched, short sound. Either can occur with atelectasis, pleural effusion, or pneumonia. Can also can be a normal finding in patients who are obese or very muscular.

MEASURING DIAPHRAGMATIC EXCURSION

(movement during the respiratory cycle)

What you'll need:

- Marking pen
- Ruler

Proper technique:

- Tell the patient to take several deep breaths and hold the last exhalation.
- Begin at the top of one scapula and percuss downward on the patient's back along the scapular line until you hear resonance change to dullness when you reach the diaphragm (Figure 6-5).
- Mark this point lightly with a pen, and then repeat the same process on the other side. (Remember that the diaphragm is somewhat higher on the right side because the liver displaces it.)
- Tell the patient to take several additional deep breaths and hold the last inhalation. Repeat your percussion process and mark the diaphragm again.
- Measure the difference between the two marks on each side (Figure 6-6). A difference of 3–5 cm between the two marks on each side of the body is normal. The distance diminishes in patients with restrictive pulmonary disorders, while phrenic nerve damage can affect excursion on only one side.

FIGURE 6-5.

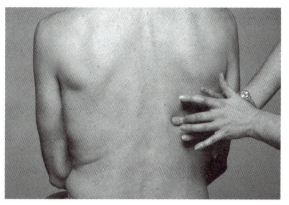

FIGURE 6-6.

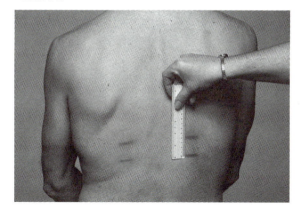

82 RN'S POCKET ASSESSMENT GUIDE

FIGURE 6-7. LOCATING THE LOBES.

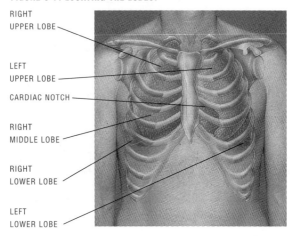

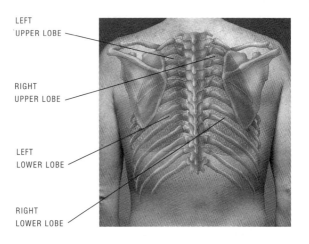

ASSESSING BREATH SOUNDS

What you'll need:

- Stethoscope

Proper technique:

- After instructing the patient to breathe through his mouth slowly, deeply, and regularly, begin auscultating the upper lobes of the lung at the apex, just above the clavicle.
- Assess systematically, moving from side to side and gradually progressing down the front until about the level of the sixth rib. Keep in mind that some lung sounds will be blocked by the heart and breasts.
- To auscultate the lower lobes, follow a similar pattern on the patient's back, remaining just next to the spine until you reach below the scapulae. Then move out from along the spine to the scapular lines until just above the 10th rib.
- Once you've listened along the back, auscultate the right and left sides to assess portions of the lower lobes not easily reached from the back.
- Always be aware of the possibility of—and try to eliminate—sources of interference: The rubbing of chest hairs or clothing against the diaphragm of the stethoscope, or the brush of tubing against the side rails of the bed, can mimic abnormal breath sounds.

What you'll hear:

Normal breath sounds

BRONCHIAL	Harsh, high-pitched, loud sounds normally heard over the trachea. Expiratory phase is longer than inspiratory phase. When present in the peripheral lung fields, may indicate pneumonia.
BRONCHOVESICULAR	A combination of bronchial and vesicular sounds. Medium pitch and intensity. Inspiratory and expiratory phases are of equal duration. Normally heard at first and second intercostal spaces at left and right sternal borders, below clavicles anteriorly and between scapulae posteriorly. When heard over peripheral lung fields, may indicate early pulmonary disease.
VESICULAR	Heard over most of the peripheral lung fields. Soft, low-pitched, and heard best in the back. Inspiratory phase is longer; the expiratory phase sounds much softer and is often inaudible.

NOTE: Increased normal breath sounds are found when lung density is increased, such as with pneumonia or compression of the lung. Decreased or absent breath sounds occur when airways are obstructed with a mucous plug or foreign body, with hyperinflation of the lungs caused by emphysema or asthma, with pneumothorax, or with pleural effusion.

Abnormal (adventitious) breath sounds

CONDITION	WHAT IT SOUNDS LIKE	WHAT IT CAN MEAN
CRACKLES (RALES)	Popping noises, heard most often during inspiration. (Because they occur in brief bursts, they are labeled discontinuous.)	Fluid, pus, or mucus in the smaller airways
Fine crackles	Soft and high-pitched. Sound like the fizz of a carbonated beverage or hair being rubbed between two fingers.	May occur normally in the elderly or during shallow respirations—e.g., upon awakening or during periods of immobility. When you hear them, instruct the patient to cough and breathe deeply, then auscultate again—they may have cleared.
Medium crackles	Louder and lower-pitched	Pulmonary edema, pulmonary fibrosis, or pneumonia
Coarse crackles	Moist-sounding	Same as above
WHEEZES (SIBILANT WHEEZES)	High-pitched, and musical. May be heard during inspiration and expiration.	An asthma attack or bronchospasm

(Continued)

CONDITION	WHAT IT SOUNDS LIKE	WHAT IT CAN MEAN
RHONCHI (SONOROUS WHEEZES)	Deeper-pitched and coarser than wheezes. Audible predominantly during expiration.	Bronchitis or pneumonia
STRIDOR	Loud, musical noise that can be heard without a stethoscope. NOTE: Stridor may be almost inaudible in patients who are sedated and comatose. To detect it, place the stethoscope on the trachea just below and to the side of the Adam's apple.	Partial upper airway obstruction. Common in croup and epiglottis. Requires immediate intervention.
PLEURAL FRICTION RUB	Harsh, grating noise that sounds like a squeaky shoe or creaking floor boards. Is usually heard during inspiration, though it may occur during expiration as well.	Any condition that produces pleural irritation, including pneumonia, pulmonary infarction, tumors, and pleural effusion.

If you detect abnormal breath sounds, continue to listen in that area and instruct the patient to say "ninety-nine." Listen for these findings:

CONDITION	WHAT IT SOUNDS LIKE	WHAT IT CAN MEAN
BRONCHOPHONY	Words sound louder and clearer than they usually do	Consolidation Atelectasis
WHISPERED PECTORILOQUY	Whispered sounds are louder and clearer than normal	Consolidation Pleural effusion

Ask the patient to say "ee" and listen for:

EGOPHONY	"ee" sound is transmitted as "ay"	Consolidation

Lastly, be alert for the following:

MEDIASTINAL CRUNCH	Though not a breath sound, this coarse, cracking vibration coincides with the heartbeat rather than respiration.	Indicates air in the mediastinum. Can accompany chest trauma and cardiopulmonary disease, or can follow CPR.

DOCUMENTING YOUR FINDINGS

- Note location of sound (e.g., which lobe(s), how far up the affected lobe).
- Note whether sound occurs during inspiration or expiration.

CHAPTER SEVEN

Cardiac system

With heart disease America's number one killer, it's hard to overemphasize the importance of a thorough cardiac examination. It begins long before you apply a stethoscope to a patient's chest—with a routine skin inspection or pulse check, for example. When you do use the stethoscope, the accuracy of your assessment depends on recognizing subtle differences between heart sounds.

SYSTEM REVIEW SHOULD COVER:

- Pain
- High blood pressure
- Palpitations
- Shortness of breath with exertion
- Shortness of breath when lying flat
- Sudden shortness of breath while sleeping
- Edema
- Syncope
- History of heart attack
- Rheumatic fever
- Heart murmur
- Last EKG
- Other tests for heart function

SPECIFIC QUESTIONS TO ASK:

- What is the nature of the chest pain or discomfort? Is it dull, sharp, stabbing, or cramping?
- How long does the pain last? What precipitates it (e.g., exercise, a stressful event)? What relieves it?
- Where does it hurt? (Ask the patient to show you.) Does the pain radiate to other parts of the body?
- Have you had this type of pain before?
- Have you had difficulty breathing? Shortness of breath?
- Have you experienced palpitations, dizziness, or fainting?
- Do you take any prescription or over-the-counter medications?
- Have you ever had a heart attack?
- Do you have hypertension, an irregular heart rhythm, cardiac disease, or leg swelling?

PHYSICAL SIGNS OF CARDIAC DISORDERS

ASSESSMENT FINDING	SIGNIFICANCE
MARFAN'S SYNDROME A hereditary condition marked by excessive height, arms that are disproportionately long in relation to the trunk, long, slender fingers, an abnormally depressed or protruding sternum, and a gaunt appearance	Can cause cardiac arrhythmias, aortic aneurysm, mitral valve insufficiency, and bacterial endocarditis
ARCUS SENILIS A light-colored ring surrounding the iris of the eye	Frequently seen in people over age 50. May indicate hereditary hypercholesterolemia or be related to ocular defects.
DE MUSSET'S SIGN A noticeable jerking of the head with each heart beat	Occurs in patients with severe aortic insufficiency
DIAGONAL BILATERAL CREASES OR FOLDS IN THE EARLOBES	Have been linked to coronary artery disease by some researchers
XANTHELASMAS Small, flat, yellowish nodules on the eyelids or the skin around the eye that are filled with cholesterol	May signal an underlying lipid disorder
SPLINTER HEMORRHAGES Red or brown longitudinal streaks in the nail beds	Seen in subacute bacterial endocarditis

(Continued)

ASSESSMENT FINDING	SIGNIFICANCE
CLUBBING OF THE FINGERS AND TOES The normal 160° angle of the nail bed and cutical often exceeds 180°.	Caused by chronic hypoxemia
EDEMA Usually in the feet and ankles but can appear around the sacrum if the patient has been lying down for a long time	Typical in right-sided heart failure; usually worsens throughout the day

FINDING THE PMI

After taking the history proceed to the examination, which should take place in a private, quiet, warm room. Have the patient lie flat. If this position is uncomfortable, elevate the head of the bed 45°.

If you are right-handed, you will be able to observe and palpate more easily if you stand at the patient's right side. The light should come from the left side so that it accentuates shadows.

Proper technique:

- Expose the chest and look for the point of maximum impulse (PMI). Usually located in the fifth left intercostal space at the midclavicular line (the mitral area), the PMI is the spot where the left ventricle lies so close to the surface that it visibly pulsates against the skin during systole.
- If the patient has large breasts that interfere with inspection, move the left breast upward or to the side, or ask the patient to do so.
- If you can't see the PMI, move the patient onto his or her left side; this often accentuates the impulse and makes it more visible.
- Gently palpate the mitral area with two fingers. Normally, the PMI covers a space 1–2 cm in diameter and feels like a light tap.

ASSESSMENT FINDING	WHAT IT CAN MEAN
PMI not detectable or barely noticeable	Hypovolemia Pericardial effusion Non-cardiac conditions such as obesity or extreme musculature
Impulse feels more forceful than usual, is felt over a greater area, or is felt in more than one intercostal space	Left ventricular hypertrophy May also occur normally in very thin people
Impulse is displaced laterally toward the axilla NOTE: Moving the patient onto his left side will displace the PMI to the left, though usually not beyond the midclavicular line.	Left ventricular hypertrophy Right-sided MI Non-cardiac problems such as pregnancy and chest deformities

After you've located the PMI:

Check other areas of the heart for pulsations and thrills—vibrations that feel like a cat's purr. Note their location. An impulse felt near the left sternal border, for example, may signal right ventricular hypertrophy.

FIGURE 7-1. THE CARDIAC CYCLE.

(A) During diastole, blood flows into the ventricles; the tricuspid and mitral valves open. (B) At the beginning of systole, the tricuspid and mitral valves snap shut, resulting in the first heart sound, S_1.

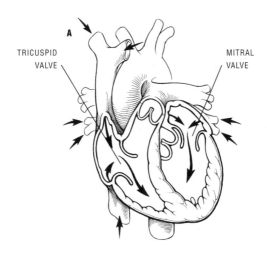

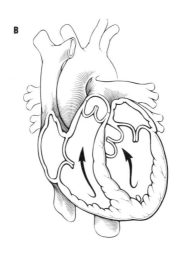

(C) During systole, the pulmonic and aortic valves open, and blood is ejected from the ventricles. (D) At the beginning of diastole, the pulmonic and aortic valves snap shut, producing the second heart sound, S_2.

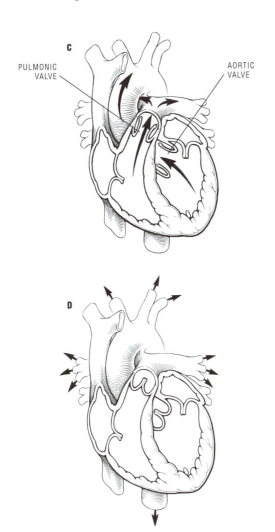

96 RN'S POCKET ASSESSMENT GUIDE

FIGURE 7-2. The five locations for cardiac auscultation are superimposed here over the heart and rib cage. When performing your assessment, either begin at the base of the heart—point 1—and proceed downwards through the next four, or start at the apex—point 5—and work back up.

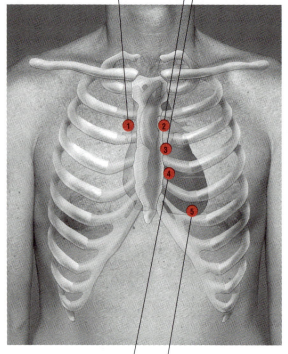

ASSESSING HEART SOUNDS

What you'll need:

- Stethoscope

Proper technique:

- Listen to the heart's rhythm and count the number of beats for one minute. Rhythm should be regular and the rate between 60 and 100.
- Note any irregularities, then listen more closely for the basic heart sounds.
- Listen first with the diaphragm, then repeat the sequence with the bell.
- Place the diaphragm firmly against the skin to hear S_1 and S_2, the normal heart sounds.
- Place the bell gently on the skin for S_3 and S_4, extra heart sounds; stretching the skin taut will change the acoustics.

98 RN'S POCKET ASSESSMENT GUIDE

What you'll listen for:

S_1 to S_4

SOUND: S_1

WHERE IT'S MOST AUDIBLE
Apex (mitral area); louder than S_2 in the tricuspid area

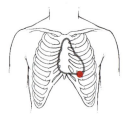

WHAT YOU'LL HEAR
Caused by the closing of the mitral and tricuspid valves, S_1 is the "lub" that's normally heard at the beginning of systole. Place the stethoscope over the mitral area and palpate the pulse; S_1 and the carotid pulse are usually synchronous. S_1 may be split—heard as two sounds clumped together—either normally or in the presence of right bundle branch block. Splitting occurs when mitral valve closure is followed rapidly by tricuspid valve closure.

SOUND: S_2

WHERE IT'S MOST AUDIBLE
Base (aortic area); louder than S_1 in the pulmonic area

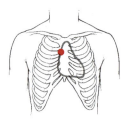

WHAT YOU'LL HEAR
Caused by the closing of the pulmonic and aortic valves, S_2 is the "dub" that normally signals the onset of diastole. May be split when aortic valve closure is followed rapidly by pulmonic valve closure. S_2 is more commonly heard as a split sound than S_1, and is usually normal.

SOUND: S_3 (VENTRICULAR GALLOP)

WHERE IT'S MOST AUDIBLE
Apex, best heard with patient on his left side

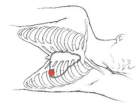

WHAT YOU'LL HEAR
Caused by blood flowing rapidly into a distended ventricle, S_3 is a dull, low-pitched "plop" that comes just after S_2 ("lub-dub-plop"). May signal the onset of congestive heart failure hours before your hear crackles (rales) in the bases of the lungs. Normal in children and young adults.

SOUND: S_4 (ATRIAL GALLOP)

WHERE IT'S MOST AUDIBLE
Apex, best heard with patient on his left side

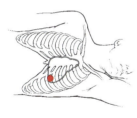

WHAT YOU'LL HEAR
Caused by blood being ejected into a stiff ventricle, S_4 is a dull, low-pitched sound heard just before S_1. May indicate MI, angina, cardiomyopathy, or stenotic valves.

Clicks, snaps, and rubs

SOUND: CLICK

WHERE IT'S MOST AUDIBLE	WHAT YOU'LL HEAR
Apex	High-pitched, extrasystolic sound, usually caused by mitral valve prolapse. May be louder during inspiration.

SOUND: PROSTHETIC VALVE CLICK

WHERE IT'S MOST AUDIBLE	WHAT YOU'LL HEAR
Location depends on which valve has been replaced.	Sound varies with type of device implanted. Often audible without a stethoscope.

SOUND: SNAP

WHERE IT'S MOST AUDIBLE	WHAT YOU'LL HEAR
Apex near the lower left sternal border	High-pitched sound heard in early diastole. Usually occurs with a thickened or stenosed mitral valve or, rarely, tricuspid valve.

SOUND: PERICARDIAL FRICTION RUB

WHERE IT'S MOST AUDIBLE	WHAT YOU'LL HEAR
Apex, with patient sitting and leaning forward	Short, scratchy noise resembling sound of creaking leather, occurring in pericarditis, MI, and after cardiac surgery. Louder with inspiration but—unlike a pleural rub—can be heard even when patient holds his breath.

Murmurs

Murmurs indicate a problem with the opening of a valve because of stiffness (stenosis), or difficulty with a valve closing because of incompetence (insufficiency, also known as regurgitation). They're grouped according to when they occur during the cardiac cycle. You'll hear murmurs associated with mitral and tricuspid valve stenosis best with a bell. The others listed here can be auscultated with the diaphragm.

Systolic murmurs

SOUND: AORTIC STENOSIS

WHERE IT'S MOST AUDIBLE
Second right intercostal space; sound may radiate to neck or left sternal border.

WHAT YOU'LL HEAR
Medium-pitched, often harsh, grating sound, occurring at mid-systole, most often with rheumatic heart disease and congenital valve disorders. Intensifies when patient squats or lies flat.

SOUND: PULMONIC STENOSIS

WHERE IT'S MOST AUDIBLE
Second or third left intercostal space; sound radiates toward the shoulder and neck.

WHAT YOU'LL HEAR
Also medium-pitched, mid-systolic, and often harsh sound, louder on inspiration and when patient is supine. Generally heard in congenital valve disease.

SOUND: MITRAL INSUFFICIENCY

WHERE IT'S MOST AUDIBLE
Apex; fifth intercostal space, left midclavicular line; sound may radiate to left axilla and back.

WHAT YOU'LL HEAR
High-pitched, blowing sound occurring throughout systole, common in rheumatic heart disease and after rupture of a ventricle's papillary muscle. Worsens during expiration and when patient is supine or on left side.

SOUND: TRICUSPID INSUFFICIENCY

WHERE IT'S MOST AUDIBLE
Lower left sternal border; sound may radiate to right sternum.

WHAT YOU'LL HEAR
Also high-pitched, blowing and holosystolic, heard in right ventricular failure and rheumatic heart disease. Intensifies on inspiration and when patient is supine.

Diastolic murmurs

SOUND: AORTIC INSUFFICIENCY

WHERE IT'S MOST AUDIBLE
Second right intercostal space and Erb's point; sound may radiate to left or right sternal border.

WHAT YOU'LL HEAR
High-pitched, blowing sound that increases when patient leans forward and holds breath. Heard during diastole in rheumatic and congenital heart disease, and with Marfan's syndrome. Aortic stenosis often a concurrent problem.

SOUND: PULMONIC INSUFFICIENCY

WHERE IT'S MOST AUDIBLE
Second left intercostal space; sound may radiate to left lower sternal border.

WHAT YOU'LL HEAR
High-pitched, blowing sound increases with inspiration. Usually associated with pulmonary hypertension.

SOUND: MITRAL STENOSIS

WHERE IT'S MOST AUDIBLE
Apex; fifth intercostal space, left midclavicular line; sound gets louder with patient on left side; does not radiate.

WHAT YOU'LL HEAR
Low-pitched, rumbling sound that increases with exercise, inspiration, and left lateral position. Commonly caused by rheumatic heart disease, often accompanied by opening snap.

SOUND: TRICUSPID STENOSIS

WHERE IT'S MOST AUDIBLE
Fourth left intercostal space, at sternal border.

WHAT YOU'LL HEAR
Low-pitched, rumbling sound that increases with inspiration. In patients with rheumatic heart disease, it usually occurs in combination with other valve problems.

DOCUMENTING YOUR FINDINGS

- Note the sound's location and whether it radiates. The murmur of mitral valve regurgitation, for example, can sometimes spread to the left axilla or back.
- Note the sound's duration—the length of time it's heard during the cardiac cycle. The murmur of tricuspid valve regurgitation is holosystolic or pansystolic—occurring throughout systole—while that of pulmonic valve regurgitation is heard more briefly during diastole.
- Note where the sound is loudest (e.g., apex or base), its tone, and its pitch:
  Is it a harsh or grating tone?
  Decrescendo (a loudness progressing to softness)?
  Crescendo (begins softly and grows louder)?
  Crescendo/decrescendo (first rises, then falls)?

HOW TO GRADE MURMURS:

Grade I	Barely audible whatever the patient's position
Grade II	Faint
Grade III	Moderately loud
Grade IV	Somewhat louder, may be accompanied by a thrill
Grade V	Loud enough to be heard with the stethoscope held just above the chest wall; accompanied by thrills
Grade VI	So loud that you can hear it without a stethoscope; accompanied by thrills

CARDIAC SYSTEM 105

FIGURE 7-3. CARDIAC RHYTHMS ON AN EKG.

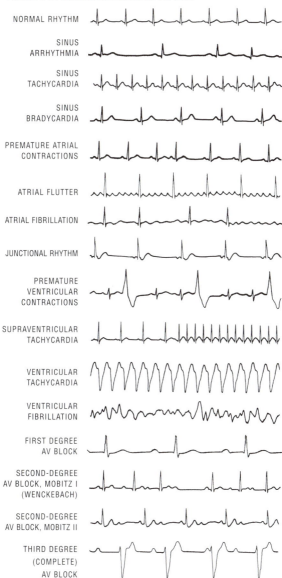

CHAPTER EIGHT

Peripheral vascular system

A careful history and physical assessment will enable you to determine if your patient is suffering from arterial or venous disease, or from a disease affecting the lymphatic vessels. Your findings may also help you distinguish peripheral vascular disease (PVD) from certain neurological disorders.

SYSTEM REVIEW SHOULD COVER:

- Pain in legs while walking
- Swelling of legs
- Varicose veins
- Thrombophlebitis
- Coolness of extremity
- Discoloration of extremity
- Loss of hair on legs
- Change in skin texture
- Ulcers

SPECIFIC QUESTIONS TO ASK:

- What is the nature of the pain or discomfort? How long does it last? What precipitates it (e.g., walking, exercise)? What relieves it (e.g., sitting, lying down)?

NOTE: Because of the risk of a pulmonary embolism in cases of deep vein thrombosis, ask patients who complain of pain in the leg about chest pain or shortness of breath. If your questions uncover a problem, refer the patient for immediate treatment.

- Is leg swelling intermittent or constant? Does it affect one leg or both?
- Do you wear tight-fitting garments or hosiery, or an abdominal binder or back brace?
- Do you now, or have you ever, smoked? If so, how many cigarettes a day and for how many years?
- Have you had any recent infections or trauma?
- Do you take any prescription or over-the-counter medications?
- Have you ever been diagnosed with hypertension, coronary artery disease, congestive heart failure, diabetes, renal disease, lupus, phlebitis, Raynaud's syndrome, or cellulitis?
- Have you ever had deep vein thrombosis, stroke, or a cerebral vascular accident?

ASSESSING LEG PAIN

ASSESSMENT FINDING	WHAT IT CAN MEAN
Leg pain aggravated by walking; relieved by rest and when legs are in dependent position.	Arterial insufficiency
Leg pain that worsens when legs are dependent; relieved by elevating legs or wearing compression stockings.	Venous insufficiency
Leg pain, usually in males, accompanied by impotence and fatigue in the hips, thighs, or calves while exercising.	Leriche's syndrome. Symptoms are caused by diminished blood flow to the pelvic arteries.
Severe leg pain, paralysis, and paresthesia. Pulse is absent in that limb and skin is pale and cold.	An acute arterial occlusion. Report it immediately; unless treated within hours, the damage may be severe and amputation may be required.
Unremitting pain after a fracture, crush injury, or peripheral vascular surgery. Pain on passive movement, which usually increases if the muscles of the affected limb are gently flexed.	Compartment syndrome. Swelling at the injury site compresses nerves and blood vessels, which in turn reduces venous flow and tissue perfusion. Most common in patients who have a cast or a wrap-around dressing.

ASSESSING FOR EDEMA, DISCOLORATION, AND ULCERS

What you'll need:

- Tape measure

MEASURE THE CIRCUMFERENCE OF EACH LEG	Suspect unilateral deep vein thrombosis, superficial thrombosis, or chronic venous insufficiency if there's a difference in circumference of 1 cm between both ankles or 2 cm between both calves. If clots have developed in both legs, however, you may see no difference in circumference because both limbs may be swollen.
CHECK BODY WEIGHT	Compare the patient's present weight against previous weight if known.
DETERMINE THE SEVERITY OF ANY EDEMA	Press down with your thumb on the dorsum of the foot for five seconds, then behind the ankle for another five. Note whether an indentation—pitting—remains in either area, and rate it using a standard rating scale. The one that follows grades edema according to how quickly the tissue bounces back after being depressed by a finger pad:

0	No fingerprint depression (non-pitting edema)
1+	1 second fingerprint depression (mild pitting edema)
2+	2 second fingerprint depression (moderate pitting)
3+	3 second fingerprint depression (severe pitting)
4+	4 second fingerprint depression (gross pitting)

CHECK FOR COLOR CHANGES

WITH ARTERIAL DISEASE:
The legs become deep red when the patient lets them hang over the side of the bed (dependent rubor). Elevating the legs for 30 seconds at a 60° angle produces pallor. Skin over the anterior tibia may be shiny and rust colored, especially in patients with diabetes. Nails are yellow and brittle, and there is little or no hair on the patient's legs or big toes.

WITH VENOUS DISEASE:
The legs have a bluish cast when the patient lets them dangle. Stasis dermatitis occurs, characterized by brown pigmentation, chronic ulcers, and flaking skin over edematous ankles; you'll usually notice it on the posterior tibial area. You may also see dilated, tortuous varicose veins.

NOTES:
1. If the patient wasn't admitted for thrombophlebitis, be particularly alert for its signs and symptoms—redness, heat, calf tenderness, and sudden unilateral edema.
2. Not all changes in skin color signal atherosclerosis or chronic venous disease. Patients who present with pain, pallor, and cyanosis in both hands or in the toes of both feet may have Raynaud's disease—arterial spasms triggered by emotional stress and cold—or Raynaud's phenomenon, which can result from frostbite, occupational trauma, or neurological disease. Once the spasm stops, the rush of blood back into ischemic tissue causes rubor.

CHECK FOR ULCERS

WITH ARTERIAL DISEASE:
Ulceration usually occurs in the toes first. Sores are generally painful, pale, circular, covered with crusts, and seen over bony prominences. If circulation to the area is severely impaired, the edges of the wound or the tip of the toes may be black. (In diabetic neuropathy, you may find ulcers at pressure points on the feet. They may or may not have crusts, but nerve degeneration often blunts the sensation of pain.)

WITH VENOUS DISEASE:
Ulcers are generally found at the ankle, where fragile, edematous skin can become traumatized. Unlike most arterial ulcers, they develop slowly and painlessly, and they're generally pink rather than black, with red, irregular margins. The surface of the ulcer is moist.

PALPATING FOR CAPILLARY REFILL, TEMPERATURE, AND PULSES

What you'll need:

- Gloves for palpating near the groin

CHECK CAPILLARY REFILL TIME
(the number of seconds it takes for color to return to a toe or fingernail bed after blanching)

A capillary refill time longer than three seconds suggests slowed peripheral perfusion and possible arterial disease. (If a yellow or thickened nail prevents assessment, note refill time for the surrounding tissue.) Also check for refill symmetry. A discrepancy in refill time between the left and right hands or feet, for instance, may indicate a blockage in the vessels feeding one side of the body.

ESTIMATE SKIN TEMPERATURE	Palpate the arms and legs with the backs of your hands. Check both paired limbs at the same time, then cross your hands and check again. (Switching hands makes any difference between the two more immediately obvious.) In arterial insufficiency, the limbs are cooler than normal. In venous disease, they are warm.
CHECK PERIPHERAL PULSES	Palpate with the pads of three fingertips but not the thumb; since your own pulse is so strong in the thumb, you may not be able to feel the patient's. Note the presence or absence, symmetry (lack of symmetry suggests impaired unilateral circulation), and volume of pulses. (Don't count the number of beats per minute; that's best done when you assess the heart.) Rate the peripheral pulse using a standard scale, such as the following:

0	Absent
1+	Weak
2+	Strong
3+	Bounding

CHECK PEDAL PULSES	Palpate these pulses on both sides of the body simultaneously. If you're unable to feel the pulse, use a Doppler. Keep in mind that a bilaterally nonpalpable pedal pulse may be normal in some people.

PERIPHERAL VASCULAR SYSTEM 115

FIGURE 8-1. SITES OF PERIPHERAL PULSES.

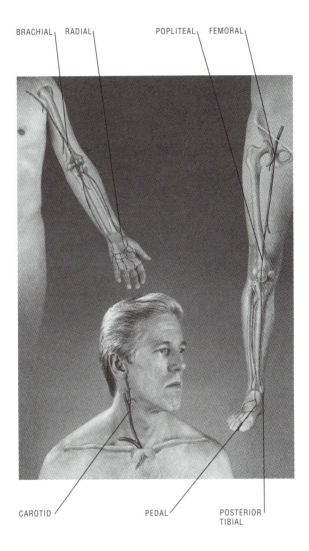

CHECK POSTERIOR TIBIAL PULSES	Palpate these pulses behind the inside of the ankles. In young adults, an absent posterior tibial pulse may be normal, but in patients over age 60 the absence of this pulse strongly suggests peripheral arterial disease.
CHECK POPLITEAL PULSES	Flex the patient's legs but tell him not to raise them in an attempt to assist you, since doing so tenses the muscles and makes palpation more difficult. Because the popliteal pulse is very deep, use both hands to apply firm pressure behind the knee, one side at a time.
CHECK FEMORAL PULSES	Since you'll be working near the groin, put on gloves. Instruct the patient to lie flat and then assess presence, volume, and symmetry of the right and left pulses. Check for an exaggerated, widened pulse, which may be a symptom of a femoral aneurysm.
	Next, palpate the radial and femoral pulses on the same side of the body at the same time. They should occur simultaneously, as do the other pulses, or the femoral should precede the radial. A delayed femoral pulse suggests aortic stenosis. (That suspicion will be supported if you discover that the patient's

PERIPHERAL VASCULAR SYSTEM 117

FIGURE 8-2. ASSESSING THE POPLITEAL PULSE.

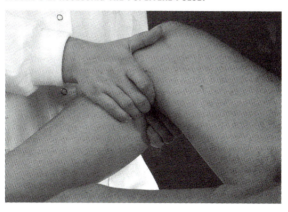

FIGURE 8-3. PALPATING THE RADIAL AND FEMORAL PULSES.

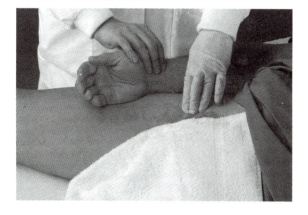

	blood pressure is lower in the legs than it is in the arms. A difference in blood pressure, however, may also suggest the possibility of a dissecting aortic aneurysm.)
CHECK RADIAL AND BRACHIAL PULSES	Palpate both radial pulses, then move up the arm to the brachials. To palpate the brachial pulses, position the pads of the fingertips just above each antecubital fossa and medial to the biceps tendon. If you press firmly, you will also be able to assess the resiliency of the artery. Normal arteries feel elastic; diseased vessels become stiff and tortuous.
CHECK CAROTID PULSES	Check these pulses one at a time so you do not impair circulation to the brain. Palpate the pulse near the base of the neck so that you don't stimulate the carotid sinus and slow the heart rate. If you have trouble finding the carotid pulse, turn the patient's head to the side to relax the adjacent sternocleidomastoid muscle.
	Immediately report any abnormalities detected in the carotid pulses.

Arterial vs. venous insufficiency

This chart summarizes the differences between the two types of peripheral vascular disease. Some patients may have both arterial and venous insufficiencies, and thus signs of both may be apparent, or signs of one may mask the other.

Characteristic	*Arterial disease*	*Venous disease*
SKIN CHANGES	Pallor, dependent rubor; skin shiny and rust-colored over front of tibia	Legs bluish when dependent, brown pigmentation at ankles; flaky dermatitis over edematous tissue
SKIN TEMPERATURE	Cool	Warm
CAPILLARY REFILL	> 3 seconds	$\leq$ 3 seconds unless perfusion impaired by severe edema
PULSES	Weak or absent	Strong and symmetrical; may be difficult to palpate pedal and posterior tibial pulses because of edema
HAIR	Absent or scant on big toe and legs	Present
EDEMA	Absent	Present, especially around ankle
ULCERS	Develop at pressure points and on toes; scab over rapidly; may be necrotic	Develop slowly over ankle; ulcer surface moist
NECROSIS (e.g., gangrene, black ulcers)	Likely	Unlikely
PAIN	Lessens with rest and when limb dependent	Lessens when limb elevated, worsens when dependent

AUSCULTATING BLOOD PRESSURE AND BRUITS

What you'll need:

- Stethoscope
- Blood pressure cuff(s)

Normal blood pressure readings may vary as much as 10–20 mm Hg from one arm to the other. A wider gap may suggest vascular insufficiency and should be reported. However, a gap of 20 mm Hg or more could also indicate a subclavian stenosis or steal, which is frequently asymptomatic and needs no treatment. To be safe, though, refer the patient for further examination.

Proper technique:

- The patient's arm should be bent and resting at heart level.
- Use a cuff that covers two-thirds of the upper arm and is neither too tight nor too loose. Keep the lower edge of the cuff one inch above the antecubital fossa.
- Palpate the brachial pulse as you inflate the BP cuff. Continue to inflate the cuff to 30 mm Hg above the point at which you no longer feel the pulse. This gives you an estimate of systolic BP and avoids an auscultatory gap often found in hypertensive patients; these gaps are usually not more than 30 mm.
- Place the stethoscope over the brachial pulse and slowly deflate the cuff. Note the systolic pressure reading as soon as you hear the first pulsation of blood entering the arteries. (If the patient has COPD, constrictive pericarditis, or pericardial effusion, this reading may drop by 10 mm Hg or more when he inhales.)
- As the mercury drops and the sound becomes more muffled, note the reading when you hear the last sound, the diastolic pressure.

Blood pressure readings in the legs are usually 10 mm Hg higher than arm readings. A smaller difference may signal arterial disease. To measure blood pressure in the legs:

- Have the patient lie on his back; apply a wide, long cuff to the lower third of the thigh, making certain that you keep the lower edge of the cuff about an inch above the knee. Listen at the popliteal space to the pulse.

122 RN'S POCKET ASSESSMENT GUIDE

FIGURE 8-4. WHERE TO LISTEN FOR BRUITS.

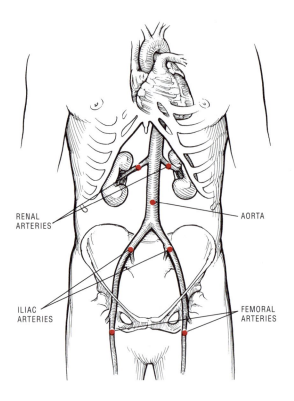

When to suspect an aneurysm:

Patients with peripheral arterial disease, especially men over 50, are particularly at risk for aneurysms, most of which occur below the renal arteries. When atherosclerosis weakens the walls of arteries in the abdomen, gentle auscultation with the bell of the stethoscope may reveal a bruit—a swishing sound caused by turbulent blood flow.

A patient with a stable aneurysm may be asymptomatic. A patient with a rapidly expanding or ruptured abdominal aortic aneurysm may have:

- A midline, pulsating mass with lateral expansion
- Mottled or bluish red skin below the waist
- Absent leg pulses
- Abdominal pain
- No urinary output

CHECKING OTHER VASCULAR PROBLEMS

CHECK FOR OCCLUSION OF THE RADIAL AND ULNAR ARTERIES

Do the Allen test on each hand: Have the patient make a tight fist to draw blood from the skin of the palm and fingers while you compress both of the arteries. If the palm does not return to its normal pink color when the patient opens his fist and you release the ulnar artery, blood flow in the ulnar artery is diminished. Similarly, if releasing only the radial artery does not return the palm color to normal, then the radial artery may be occluded.

CHECK FOR VARICOSITIES *(caused by incompetent valves in the vein)*	Perform the manual compression test: Position the fingertips of one hand firmly over the uppermost section of a suspected varicosity and then place the fingertips of the other hand 20 cm below the section. If the valves are incompetent, compressing the upper section of the vein will produce backward, turbulent blood flow that your lower hand will feel as an impulse or as a "buzzing" sensation.
CHECK HOMANS' SIGN	Flex the foot back. About half of patients with venous thrombosis will complain of deep calf pain when you do so. However, a positive Homans' sign can also indicate an inflamed calf muscle.

ASSESSING THE LYMPHATIC SYSTEM

Palpate the various clusters of lymph nodes for size, shape, mobility, consistency, and tenderness. Normally, lymph nodes are not palpable; when they are, think infection or malignancy.

Start with the nodes in the head and neck, then move on to the nodes in the arms and trunk. A breast examination should include palpating the central axillary, infraclavicular, pectoral, and subscapular nodes that drain portions of the chest, sides, and back.

Finally, assess lymphatic drainage of the groin and legs. The inguinal nodes drain the lower abdomen, the buttocks, part of the thighs, and the genitals, and the femoral nodes drain the low thighs, calves, and feet.

PERIPHERAL VASCULAR SYSTEM 125

FIGURE 8-5. THE LYMPHATIC SYSTEM.

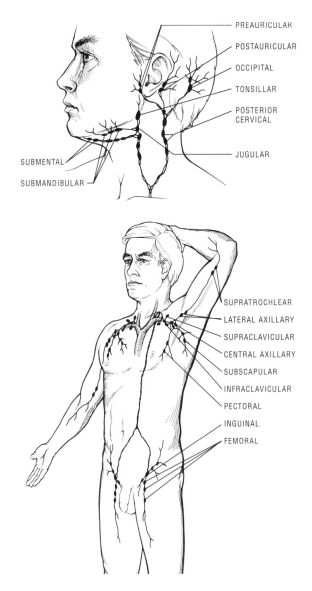

ASSESSMENT FINDING	WHAT IT CAN MEAN
Hard, fixed nodes	Metastatic cancer or lymphoma, such as Hodgkin's disease. An enlarged left supraclavicular node, for example, may be an early sign of abdominal cancer.
Swollen, tender nodes in only one area	Injury or infection in the tissues as they drain
Persistent generalized lymphadenopathy—lymph nodes that remain enlarged for at least three months and are found in at least two places besides the groin	AIDS or another severe infectious disease
Small, rubbery, non-tender nodes that resemble buckshot	The aftermath of a local infection; no clinical significance

CHAPTER NINE

Gastrointestinal system

When your patient has GI distress, a thorough abdominal assessment is in order, including a rectal exam. Given the wealth of organs, blood vessels, and glands in the abdomen, pinpointing the exact location of your patient's problem requires a systematic, quadrant by quadrant approach.

Remember, when assessing the abdomen, the usual progression of inspection, palpation, percussion, and auscultation changes. To prevent distortion of bowel sounds caused by pressing on the abdomen, you'll move from inspection directly to auscultation.

SYSTEM REVIEW SHOULD COVER:

- Appetite
- Excessive hunger
- Excessive thirst
- Nausea
- Swallowing
- Constipation
- Diarrhea
- Heartburn
- Vomiting
- Abdominal pain
- Change in stool color
- Change in stool caliber
- Change in stool consistency
- Frequency of bowel movements
- Vomiting blood (hematemesis)
- Rectal bleeding (hematochezia)
- Black, tarry stools
- Weakness
- Fatigue
- Shortness of breath
- Laxative or antacid use or abuse
- Excessive belching
- Food intolerance
- Change in abdominal girth
- Hemorrhoids
- Infections
- Jaundice
- Rectal pain
- Previous abdominal X-ray
- Hepatitis
- Liver disease
- Gallbladder disease
- Pancreatitis

SPECIFIC QUESTIONS TO ASK:

- Are you presently in pain? On a scale of one to 10 with 10 being the worst, how bad is it?
- Have you had indigestion in the past 24 hours?
- During the past 24 hours, has your diet included anything you could be allergic to?
- Do you belch, have excessive gas, or experience nausea, vomiting, or diarrhea?
- When and how often do symptoms occur? What precipitates them and what, if anything, relieves them?

- Have you been experiencing any weakness or fatigue? (Can occur with GI bleeding.)
- Have you had any shortness of breath? (Can occur with GI bleeding or ascites.)
- Do you drink alcohol? If so, how often and how much? Do you have a history of alcohol abuse?
- Do you take any prescription or over-the-counter medications?
- Have you had any recent falls or abdominal trauma?
- Have you recently noticed any changes in your appetite or weight?
- Do you wear dentures? Do you have chewing or swallowing difficulties?
- Have you traveled recently? Is so, where?
- How frequently do you have a bowel movement? What's the color, amount, and consistency of the stool?
- Do you have rectal bleeding, hemorrhoids, or pain on defecation?
- Have you ever had, or do you now have, ulcers, ulcerative colitis, Crohn's disease, diverticulitis, hepatitis, pancreatitis, or cirrhosis of the liver?
- Have you or a family member ever had cancer?

ASSESSING CONTOUR, MOVEMENT, AND SKIN

Before starting the exam, ask the patient to empty his bladder. Then have him lie on his back, arms at his sides, with knees flexed to relax the abdomen. You can put pillows under his head and knees if he's more comfortable that way.

INSPECT CONTOUR	Note whether the abdomen is flat, convex (rounded), or concave. Note any asymmetric distention or protrusion, which could indicate hernia, tumor, enlarged organs, or bowel obstruction.
OBSERVE SURFACE MOVEMENT	You may see a slight pulsation of the aorta at the epigastrium, which is normal. Note any visible peristaltic movement; it could indicate intestinal obstruction, in which case you'll see a hyperperistaltic wave above the obstructed area.
INSPECT SKIN	Note color, texture, hydration, and any lesions or unusual markings, including moles, warts, rashes, petechiae, and keloids. Red-blue or purple striae could mean liver disease or Cushing's syndrome. Spider angiomas—small distended capillaries that radiate from a central point—could indicate hepatic failure. Cullen's sign, a circular blue discoloration of the umbilicus, may be a sign of intraperitoneal bleeding or acute hemorrhagic pancreatitis.
ASSESS STOMA	Note its shape and color. It should protrude slightly from the abdomen and have the same moistness and reddish-pink tint as the inside of the mouth. Skin around the site should be free of redness and irritation.

GASTROINTESTINAL SYSTEM **131**

FIGURE 9-1. MAPPING THE ABDOMEN.

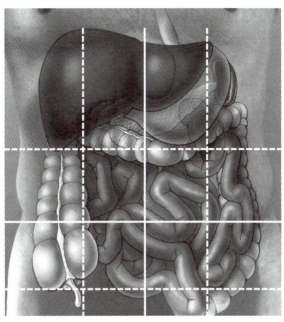

AUSCULTATING ABDOMINAL SOUNDS

For most clinical purposes, you'll divide the abdomen into four quadrants, as shown above. Draw imaginary lines from the sternum to the symphysis pubis and across the umbilicus. If a more detailed examination is called for, use the nine-segment grid also illustrated here.

What you'll need:

- Stethoscope

TIP:

- Warm the stethoscope diaphragm to help prevent guarding when you examine the patient.

AUSCULTATE BOWEL SOUNDS

Place the stethoscope over each quadrant and listen for the clicks and gurgles that normally occur five to 35 times per minute. If after five minutes you don't hear anything in one quadrant, move on to the next.

If bowel sounds are present note their character and frequency. Bowel sounds are considered hyperactive if they occur every two to three seconds, and hypoactive if no more than one occurs per minute. Borborygmi—loud, prolonged rumbling noises—are caused by the movement of gas, and can be an early sign of bowel obstruction. Decreased or absent bowel sounds may point to peritonitis or ileus. Diarrhea or an intestinal obstruction in its early stages can increase bowel sounds, but they decrease as the obstruction worsens.

AUSCULTATE VASCULAR SOUNDS

Use the stethoscope's bell to auscultate vascular sounds over the abdominal aorta and the right and left renal arteries, located near the epigastrium and right and left upper quadrants. In the lower quadrants, auscultate the iliac and femoral arteries. If the patient has an abdominal aneurysm, you may hear a bruit—the swishing sound of turbulent blood flow.

GASTROINTESTINAL SYSTEM **133**

	CAUTION: If you hear a bruit, do not percuss or palpate the abdomen, as this may cause the aneurysm to rupture.
AUSCULTATE FOR FRICTION RUBS	Listen at the right and left upper quadrants for friction rubs over the liver and spleen. These grating sounds may indicate a hepatic tumor, splenic infarct, or inflammation of the peritoneum.

PERCUSSING THE ABDOMEN

Begin by percussing each quadrant to get an overview of sounds. Then percuss specific structures.

What you'll need:

■ Marking pen   ■ Tape measure

WHAT YOU'LL HEAR:	**WHERE YOU'LL HEAR IT:**
DULLNESS—a medium-pitched sound, like a thud, of medium duration.	Over solid organs, tumors, and fluid.
TYMPANY—a high-pitched, hollow sound, like a drum beat, of medium duration.	Over air-filled organs.
CHECK LIVER SIZE	With the patient lying on his back, begin percussing at the right midclavicular line at the level of the umbilicus and move upward. The sound should change from tympany to dullness when you reach the lower border of the organ's

right lobe. Mark that spot with a marking pen. Find its upper border by percussing from about the third intercostal space down to the point of dullness, and mark that spot as well. The distance between the marks should be between 6 and 12 cm. More than 12 cm suggests hepatomegaly—a common finding in cirrhosis.

CHECK FOR THE SPLEEN	Have the patient remain supine. Percuss at the lowest intercostal space along the left anterior midaxillary line. If the spleen is enlarged, the normally tympanic sound will change to dullness when the patient takes a deep breath.
CHECK FOR KIDNEY TENDERNESS	Do gentle fist percussion: Have the patient sit up. Approach him from behind and put the ball of your left hand at the costovertebral angle that forms where the 11th and 12th ribs meet the spine. Strike your open left hand with your right fist, using just enough pressure to produce a thud. If the patient has a renal infection, this blow should cause pain.
CHECK FOR ASCITES	Test for shifting dullness: With the patient on his back, percuss from flank to umbilicus, marking the point at which dullness changes to tympany. Then turn the patient on his

side and percuss the same area again. The mark will move significantly if there is fluid buildup.

Evaluate the progression of ascites by periodically measuring abdominal girth. To ensure consistency between measurements, bring the tape measure around the abdomen at the largest diameter and mark the abdomen along the tape lines.

PALPATING THE ABDOMEN

TIP:

- If your patient is ticklish, place your hand over the patient's hand and move it from place to place just to get him used to being touched. Then substitute your hand for his and begin with light palpation.

Proper technique:

LIGHT PALPATION

- Using the pads of your fingertips, start in areas you expect to be normal and progress to those where you suspect tenderness. Feel for bulges, which may indicate a hernia. If the patient tenses his abdominal muscles at your touch, suspect inflammation. Board-like rigidity throughout the abdomen suggests generalized peritonitis.

- To distinguish a tumor or a mass that's beneath the abdominal wall itself, have the patient tense his abdomen by raising his head. If the mass is under the wall, contracting the muscles will obscure it.

- Once you've located a mass, describe its size, shape, consistency, and mobility. Note whether it's tender and if it pulsates or moves when the patient breathes.

DEEP PALPATION

CAUTION: Do not perform deep palpation on areas where you noted tenderness or pulsation on light palpation.

- As you palpate, monitor the patient's facial expression for signs of discomfort. The areas over the aorta, cecum, and sigmoid colon are especially sensitive, so proceed cautiously.
- Check for rebound tenderness—the patient feels more discomfort when you release your hand than when you press down. With appendicitis, you're likely to get a positive response in the right lower quadrant at McBurney's point—about halfway between the iliac crest and the umbilicus. The left lower quadrant may be tender in left-sided ulcerative colitis.
- If an organ is palpable, note its size, shape, tenderness, and consistency.

PALPATE LIVER	Place one hand on top of the other near the right lower costal border. Have the patient breathe in, and press down and up (Figure 9-2).
	As an alternative, place both hands side by side at the right lower costal border, and hook your fingertips over the edge of the rib cage. Have the patient breath in, and press down (Figure 9-3).

GASTROINTESTINAL SYSTEM 137

FIGURE 9-2.

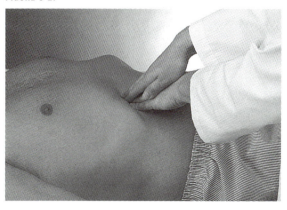

FIGURE 9-3.

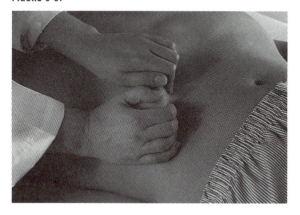

138 RN'S POCKET ASSESSMENT GUIDE

FIGURE 9-4.

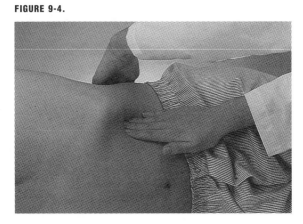

FIGURE 9-5.

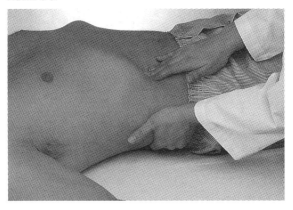

GASTROINTESTINAL SYSTEM

PALPATE SPLEEN

Have the patient lie on his right side, which will force the organ to fall forward. Standing to his right, reach over him and place your left hand on his back at the lower left costal border. Place your right hand on his anterior left lower costal border. Have the patient breathe in, and press forward and up (Figure 9-4).

CAUTION: Be extremely gentle when palpating for the spleen. It's unlikely you'll feel the organ unless it's triple its normal size, and at that point too much pressure can easily rupture it.

PALPATE KIDNEYS

A normal right kidney may or may not be palpable. With the patient lying on his back or his left side, place one hand on the patient's back between the 11th and 12th ribs. As he breathes in, use the fingertips of the other hand to palpate the anterior right upper quadrant at the midclavicular line (Figure 9-5).

With the patient lying on his back or right side, perform the same technique at the left upper quadrant to try and palpate the left kidney. The left kidney is usually not palpable because it's situated higher up in the abdomen and is thus less accessible.

CAUTION: Don't try to palpate a kidney if you know the

	patient has polycystic disease or Wilms' tumor—a type of renal cancer that is usually seen in young children—or if the patient has had a transplant. Doing so could rupture the capsule surrounding the tumor or cause bleeding.
PALPATE BLADDER/UTERUS	If you think the patient may have a distended urinary bladder or enlarged uterus, check the suprapubic area. An empty bladder and a normal, nonpregnant uterus are usually not palpable. Use a ruler and marking pen to note findings to the contrary. A distended bladder feels like a smooth, round, and tense mass.

ASSESSING THE RECTUM

Before starting the exam, ask the patient to void. Have him either bend over the examining table, assume a left lateral position on the table with hip and knees flexed, or assume a knee-to-chest position.

What you'll need:

- Gloves
- A water-soluble lubricant
- Material for guaiac testing

INSPECT PERINEUM AND PERIANAL AREAS	Place your dominant hand on the patient's hip to stabilize his position. Gently, spread the buttocks with your other hand. Inspect the perineum and perianal areas for abnormalities such as lesions hemorrhoids, inflammations, discoloration, or discharges.
PALPATE RECTUM	Apply a water-soluble lubricant to your gloved examining finger. Ask the patient to bear down in order to relax the anal sphincter, and slowly insert the ball of your finger into the rectum. Note sphincter tone. Palpate the rectal walls for lesions.
CHECK STOOL	As you withdraw your finger, inspect your glove for blood or feces. Any feces that doesn't have a brown hue is considered abnormal. Test stool (guaiac) for occult blood.

CHAPTER TEN

Genitourinary system

No other body system is more private than the GU system. Because of its personal nature, the patient may deliberately "edit" his or her history to avoid embarrassment. To elicit accurate, complete information and to assuage anxiety about the upcoming physical exam, take some time to build rapport and trust. During the assessment itself, be confident, relaxed, and unhurried. Defer sensitive questions prompted by your findings until after the exam is over.

In men, the urinary and reproductive systems are combined; in women, they are in close proximity. For both men and women, then, the health of one system impacts the other. This section focuses on the external examination of the GU system, as well as the examination for femoral and inguinal hernias. A more comprehensive assessment is customarily performed by physicians or nurse practitioners during a routine physical.

SYSTEM REVIEW SHOULD COVER:

- Urinary frequency
- Urinary urgency
- Difficulty starting the stream
- Incontinence
- Excessive urination (polyuria)
- Infrequent urination (oliguria)
- Pain on urination (dysuria)
- Burning
- Blood in urine
- Infections, including STDs
- Stones
- Bed-wetting
- Flank pain
- Awakening at night to urinate (nocturia)
- History of retention
- Urine color
- Urine odor

MALE GENITALIA:

- Lesions on penis
- Discharge
- Impotence
- Pain
- Scrotal masses
- Hernias
- Frequency of intercourse
- Problems with intercourse
- Ability to enjoy sexual relations
- Fertility problems
- Prostate problems
- History of venereal disease and treatment

FEMALE GENITALIA:

- Lesions on external genitalia
- Itching
- Discharge
- Last Pap smear and result
- Frequency of intercourse
- Pain during intercourse
- Ability to enjoy sexual relations
- Birth control methods
- Fertility problems
- Hernias
- History of venereal disease and treatment
- History of DES exposure
- Age at menarche
- Interval between menstrual periods
- Duration of menstrual periods
- Amount of flow
- Menstrual pain
- Date of last period
- Bleeding between periods
- Number of pregnancies
- Abortions
- Term deliveries
- Complications of pregnancies
- Description(s) of labor
- Number of living children
- Age at menopause
- Menopausal symptoms
- Postmenopausal bleeding

BREASTS:

- Lumps
- Discharge
- Pain
- Tenderness
- Self-examination
- Surgeries, including implants and breast reduction
- Mammogram history
- Breast disease history, self and family

SPECIFIC QUESTIONS TO ASK:

- How many times a day do you urinate?
- Is the stream strong and steady?
- Do you ever find that you can't hold your urine? If yes, when (e.g., after coughing or sneezing)?
- Do you have trouble starting your urine stream?
- Do you have any pain when urinating?
- What beverages do you drink? In what quantities? At what time?
- Do you have any allergies, particularly to shellfish or iodine?
- Do you follow a specific diet or exercise routine?
- Are you sexually active? If so, how often do you have intercourse?
- How many sexual partners have you had?
- Do you use birth control? Regularly? What type?
- Have you ever had a sexually transmitted disease?
- Have you ever had, or do you now have, cancer, hypertension, cardiac disease, kidney problems, or endocrine conditions such as diabetes, Cushing's syndrome, or Addison's disease?
- Is there any family history of urinary disorders?
- Do you now, or have you ever, smoked? If so, how many cigarettes a day and for how many years?
- Do you drink alcohol or use any illicit drugs? If so, how often?
- Do you take any prescription or over-the-counter medications?

In addition to these questions, cover the gender-specific points noted under System Review.

ASSESSING THE KIDNEYS AND BLADDER

See Chapter 9, Gastrointestinal System.

EXAMINING THE MALE GENITALIA

What you'll need:

- Gloves
- Flashlight for transillumination
- Slides and fixative spray for possible culturing
- Reflex hammer or tongue blade

TIPS:

- Keep door closed for privacy.
- Keep room temperature comfortable.
- If the patient has an erection during the exam, continue with your assessment; stopping the exam will only focus attention on the incident. You may also want to inform the patient that an erection is merely a normal physiologic reaction to the procedure.

FIGURE 10-1. THE MALE REPRODUCTIVE SYSTEM.

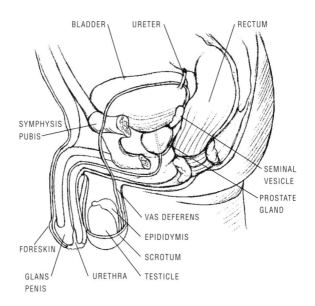

CHECK PUBIC HAIR	Look for signs of infestation (e.g., lice or scabies).
INSPECT PENIS	Note size, shape, appearance, and the presence of scars, inflammation, swelling, or lesions.
INSPECT PREPUCE (FORESKIN)	Gently retract the foreskin if present—or ask the patient to retract it himself—and check for irritation and discharge. Smegma, a white cheeselike substance, is normal. Replace the foreskin to prevent edema.
PALPATE GLANS	Gently compress the glans between your thumb and forefinger. The meatus will open. The edges should appear pink and smooth, and there should be no discharge.
INSPECT URINARY MEATUS	Look for discharge, growths, lack of cleanliness, anatomic abnormalities, and congenital displacement, either inferiorly and proximally (hypospadias) or superiorly (epispadias). If the meatus discharges, note the quantity, color, odor, and viscosity, and take a specimen for culture. If no discharge appears but the patient has a history of discharge, ask him to milk the shaft of the penis, starting at the base (or do this yourself if necessary). This should produce a discharge.
PALPATE SHAFT	With the penis between your thumb and first two fingers, palpate for masses and tenderness.

INSPECT SCROTUM

Examine the back and front surfaces for lumps, lesions, or edemas. Lumps may be due to chronic illness (congestive or renal failure), hydrocele, scrotal edema, or hernia. Sebaceous cysts—yellowy, non-tender, firm, multiple nodules about one centimeter in diameter—are common on the scrotum and are benign. A single, painless, pea-size nodule may indicate testicular cancer.

Painful swelling suggests acute epididymitis, acute orchitis, torsion of the spermatic cords (the cords run from the superior portion of the epididymis up through the inguinal canal), or inguinal hernia. Transilluminate any swelling with a flashlight: Darken the room and shine the beam behind the scrotum on the area of the mass. A red glow means the swelling contains serous fluid. Blood, tissue, tumor, and hernias will not transilluminate.

PALPATE TESTES	Gently palpate each testis and the epididymis between your thumb and first two fingers. They should feel oval, firm, and smooth, appear symmetrical (although one testicle may hang lower than the other), and be tender to the slightest touch. The scrotal contents should move easily within the sacs.
PALPATE THE SPERMATIC CORD, WHICH INCLUDES THE VAS DEFERENS	Palpate the cord between your thumb and forefinger. It should feel smooth and not be tender. Note any swelling, nodules, and veins. Multiple tortuous veins indicate a varicocele or cyst, which often also suggests the presence of a hydrocele. A thick and beaded vas deferens—the duct system used to transport sperm— suggests chronic infection.
TEST CREMASTERIC REFLEX	With the handle of the reflex hammer or a tongue blade, stroke the patient's inner thigh. The testicle and scrotum on the stroked side should rise, indicating that the L1 and L2 spinal nerves are intact.

152 RN'S POCKET ASSESSMENT GUIDE

FIGURES 10-2. FEMALE GENITALIA, INTERNAL VIEW.

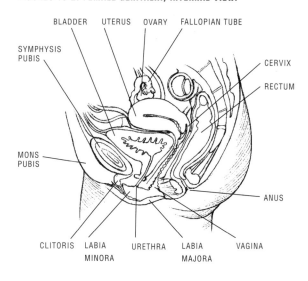

FIGURE 10-3. FEMALE GENITALIA, EXTERNAL VIEW.

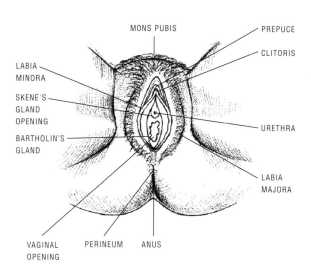

EXAMINING THE EXTERNAL FEMALE GENITALIA

Before starting the exam, ask the patient to empty her bladder. Then have her lie on her back with her knees bent and apart and her feet on the bed, or have her assume the lithotomy position on an exam table. Assist the patient as necessary. Drapery should cover her knees and thighs.

What you'll need:

- Gloves
- Movable lamp
- Slides and fixative spray for possible culturing

TIPS:

- Keep door closed for privacy.
- Keep room temperature comfortable.
- If you are male, consider summoning a female assistant.
- Since the patient won't be able to see what you're doing, tell her when you are going to begin the exam.

INSPECT PUBIC HAIR	Check for signs of infestation (e.g., lice or scabies).
INSPECT AND PALPATE THE LABIA MAJORA	Separate the labia majora with your gloved hand and look for inflammation, ulceration, swelling, nodules, and discharge. Palpate between your thumb and second finger, feeling for irregularities or nodules.
INSPECT AND PALPATE THE LABIA MINORA, CLITORIS, URETHRAL ORIFICE, VAGINAL OPENING (INTROITUS), AND PERINEUM	Note any inflammation, masses, lesions, erythema, vesicles, swelling, fissures, bleeding, discharge, or tenderness.

MILK THE URETHRA	If there is edema and erythema around the urethral meatus—indicating inflammation of the paraurethral (Skene's) glands—insert your index finger into the vagina up to the second joint of the finger. Exerting upward pressure, milk the urethra from the inside outward. Culture any discharge, which usually indicates infection.
PALPATE BARTHOLIN'S GLANDS	If there is labial swelling or redness—suggesting infection of Bartholin's glands—insert your index finger into the vagina and place your thumb outside the posterior labia majora. Palpate between the two fingers for any swelling, lesions, or tenderness. Observe for drainage from the duct opening and culture any that is present.

ASSESSING FOR HERNIA (MALES AND FEMALES)

INSPECT FEMORAL AND INGUINAL AREAS	With the patient standing, look for any bulges. Then ask the patient to bear down or cough. If a bulge appears, suspect a hernia.
PALPATE FOR INGUINAL HERNIA	**IN MEN:** Ask the patient to shift his weight to his left leg. Place your right index finger at a low point in the right side of the scrotal sac and invaginate

GENITOURINARY SYSTEM 155

FIGURE 10-4. PALPATING FOR AN INGUINAL HERNIA.

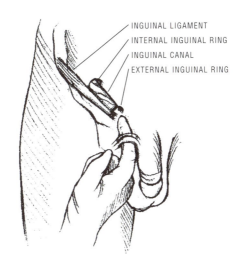

INGUINAL LIGAMENT
INTERNAL INGUINAL RING
INGUINAL CANAL
EXTERNAL INGUINAL RING

FIGURE 10-5. PALPATING FOR A FEMORAL HERNIA.

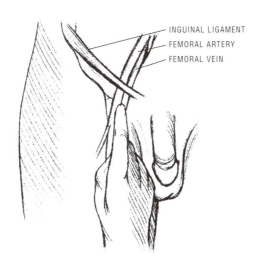

INGUINAL LIGAMENT
FEMORAL ARTERY
FEMORAL VEIN

your finger into the loose folds. Palpate up the length of the spermatic cord to the external inguinal ring; the opening of the ring will feel like a triangular slit. In some patients, you'll be able to pass your finger through the ring. If so, gently insert it into the inguinal canal.

With your finger either against the ring or in the canal, ask the patient to bear down or cough. If a hernia exists, you will feel an impulse or pushing against your finger.

Repeat the procedure on the left side of the patient's body, using your left hand.

IN WOMEN:
With the patient standing, palpate the area of the labia majora up and lateral to the inguinal region (the lower, medial portion of the abdominal wall). If there's a hernia, you will feel a bulge in the area.

PALPATE FOR FEMORAL HERNIA	**IN BOTH MEN AND WOMEN:** Place your finger on the patient's anterior thigh near the area of the femoral canal. Ask the patient to bear down or cough. Note any swelling or tenderness.

Palpate the horizontal inguinal lymph node chain along the groin, inferior to the inguinal ligament, and the vertical

	chain along the upper, inner thigh. It's normal to feel an isolated, small, movable node. Any enlargement, fixing, or hardening is abnormal.
ASSESS FOR SCROTAL HERNIA	If you suspect that a large scrotal mass may be a hernia, have the patient lie down and auscultate the mass for bowel sounds. You may be able to hear bowel sounds over a hernia; you won't hear them over a hydrocele.

IF YOUR EXAM REVEALS A HERNIA:

Have the patient lie down to see if it spontaneously disappears. If it doesn't, exert gentle pressure against the mass to try and reduce it—return it to the abdominal cavity. Do *not* do this if the patient complains of nausea, vomiting, or tenderness. The hernia may be strangulated—blood supply to the entrapped contents is compromised—and require surgery.

CHAPTER ELEVEN

Geriatric patients
Special considerations

The physiologic changes of aging alter a range of assessment parameters. The elderly are also prone to certain clinical emergencies; their homeostasis is fragile and their overall reserve is decreased. Automatically attributing abnormal clinical findings to old age can result in costly delays in treatment; initiating interventions that aren't warranted can prove just as harmful.

To perform an accurate and complete assessment, then, you need to know and consider the changes of aging. One caveat to remember: Old people differ from each other as much as young people do. Not every elderly patient will experience the changes discussed here.

CHANGES OF AGING BY SYSTEM

NEUROLOGIC	*Decreased:* Response and reaction time Number of brain cells Amount of neurotransmitters REM and Stage IV sleep
MUSCULOSKELETAL	*Decreased:* Height Muscle mass, tone, and strength Bone mass and mineralization
	Increased: Joint and cartilage erosion Thinning of vertebrae
RESPIRATORY	*Decreased:* Respiratory muscle tone Number of functional alveoli Ciliary action PO_2
	Increased: Anteroposterior diameter of chest
CARDIOVASCULAR	*Decreased:* Elasticity of heart and arteries Efficiency of heart and peripheral valves
	Increased: Formation of atherosclerotic plaques Peripheral resistance

GASTROINTESTINAL	*Decreased:* Esophageal peristalsis External sphincter reflexes Taste sensation Saliva production Liver size, weight, and efficiency Gastric acid secretion Intestinal motility
GENITOURINARY	*Decreased:* Glomerular filtration rate Renal blood flow Renal mass Nephron units Bladder muscle tone Sphincter tone
	FEMALE: Atrophic vulva Flattening of labia Vagina shorter, drier, more friable
	MALE: Testes smaller and less firm Ejaculations slower and less forceful

THE PHYSICAL ASSESSMENT: WHAT TO EXPECT

ASSESSMENT FINDING	PHYSIOLOGIC CAUSE
INTEGUMENTARY	
Skin: thin, dry, fragile, decreased turgor, increased wrinkles	Thinning of skin layers Decrease in gland activity Loss of subcutaneous fat
Injuries slow to heal	Diminished capillary flow
Decreased perspiration Lesions: seborrheic keratoses, senile angiomas, pigmentation deposits, senile keratosis, basal cell carcinoma	Decreased sweat gland activity Cellular changes Environmental injury
Nails: thickened, yellowed, and ridged	Cellular changes
NEUROLOGICAL	
Sleep disturbances; more wakeful periods, need for naps, insomnia	Stages of sleep altered Chronic or acute disorders Medication effect Decreased physical activity
Slowed reaction time Learning takes longer	Conduction deficiencies
Mild, recent memory losses or confusion	As above Reduced cerebral blood flow
Depression	Alteration in naturally occurring chemicals and hormones
TASTE AND SMELL	
Poor nutrition Decreased appetite Foods taste bland	Reduced taste buds and olfactory receptors

ASSESSMENT FINDING	PHYSIOLOGIC CAUSE
TOUCH	
Diminished sensitivity to pain, heat, pressure Diminished ability to distinguish items by touch (stereognosis)	Conduction deficiencies
VISION	
Dry eyes	Decreased tear production
Problem reading at close range	Lens hardens
Pupils slow to react to light	Diminished muscle response
Clouding of lens	Cataracts
Requires more light to see Slow adaptation to dark, poor night vision	Decreased light perception threshold
HEARING	
Speech discrimination difficulty Decreased ability to hear high-pitched sounds	Ear wax impaction Degenerative changes

ASSESSMENT FINDING	PHYSIOLOGIC CAUSE
MUSCULOSKELETAL	
Decrease in height	Weakened spinal structures Shrinking of intravertebral disks
Kyphosis	Bone demineralization
Decrease in muscle mass, tone, and strength	Decreased muscle fibers Decreased physical activity
Diminished mobility, flexibility, and range of motion	Decreased capillary circulation
Diminished balance and reaction time	Decreased innervation Decreased physical activity
Joint pain	Joint and cartilage erosion Bony overgrowths
RESPIRATORY	
Decreased breath sounds at bases Fatigue and breathlessness with sustained activity	Lung tissue loses elasticity Respiration compromised Slow cardiac response to increased oxygen demands
Decreased effectiveness of cough Difficulty coughing secretions	Reflexes diminished Decreased ciliary action
Increase in the anteroposterior diameter of the chest	Intravertebral disc collapse Costal cartilage calcification
Decreased chest expansion	Costal cartilage calcification
Decreased depth of respiration	Respiratory muscle weakness

GERIATRIC PATIENTS 165

ASSESSMENT FINDING	PHYSIOLOGIC CAUSE
CARDIOVASCULAR	
Early systolic murmur (S_4) Fatigue	Valves more rigid and thick
Premature beats and arrhythmias	Conduction deficiencies
Under conditions of stress, the pulse is slow to respond and slow to return to normal	Diminished baroreceptor response Myocardium loses elasticity
Increased systolic and diastolic blood pressures Widened pulse pressure	Blood vessels lose elasticity Peripheral resistance increases
Vascular tortuosity and prominence in the forehead, neck, and extremities Varicose veins Edema	Blood vessels lose elasticity Peripheral valves weaken Blood vessels kink Decreased activity resulting in decreased venous return
GASTROINTESTINAL	
Atrophy of gums with loss of teeth or decay	Poor dental care
Dry mouth	Decreased saliva production
Decreased appetite and thirst Early satiety Cough or choking Dysphagia Patient complains of heartburn and reflux	Diminished esophageal peristalsis Delayed emptying Gag reflex diminished Hiatal hernia
Constipation/fecal impaction Fecal incontinence	Decreased intestinal motility Decreased anal sphincter tone

ASSESSMENT FINDING	PHYSIOLOGIC CAUSE
GENITOURINARY	
Increased nocturia, frequency, and urgency	Diminished sensation, hormone response Decreased bladder capacity
Dehydration	Decreased thirst Decreased body water storage
Increased adverse and toxic effects from certain medications, dyes	Decreased renal clearance
Decreased glycosuria in diabetics	Increased renal threshold
Incontinence: urge overflow stress	Decreased bladder capacity Decreased bladder innervation Weakened musculature and sphincter tone
Males: difficulty initiating urine stream	Enlarged prostate
Females: painful intercourse, delayed orgasm	Vaginal dryness Atrophy secondary to decreased hormonal stimulation
Males: delayed erection and achievement of orgasm	Diminished hormonal and sensory cues

CHECKLIST FOR GERIATRIC EMERGENCIES

Common pathologies that bring elderly patients to the emergency department are listed below. The order of problems under each subheading roughly reflects the frequency with which they occur.

Differential for coma

TOXIC-METABOLIC DISORDERS

Drug interaction or overdose
Hypoglycemia
Diabetic ketoacidosis
Non-ketotic hyperosmolar coma
Postictal state
Sepsis
Alcohol
Wernicke's encephalopathy
Hypertensive encephalopathy
Hypoxia
Meningitis
Hepatic coma
Uremia
Hypercarbia
Hyponatremia
Hypercalcemia
Addisonian crisis
Hypothermia

NEUROSURGICAL CONDITIONS

Intracranial hematomas, tumors, and abscesses
Cerebellar hemorrhage
Subdural empyema

NEUROLOGICAL DISEASES

Cerebral hemorrhages and infarctions
Basilar occlusion
Brain stem tumor
Meningitis

Differential for temporary loss of consciousness

Embolism from coronary or other arteries
Arrhythmia
Postictal state
Hypertension
Hypoglycemia
Dehydration
Temporal arteritis
Effects of trauma (especially from a neck injury)
Blood loss
Hemiplegic migraine
Underlying blood dyscrasia

Differential for upper GI pain

Esophagitis
Gastritis
Peptic ulcer
Esophageal reflux
Hiatal hernia
Duodenitis
Varices
Mallory-Weiss tear
Cancer

Differential for abdominal pain

THORACIC CONDITIONS

Pneumonia
Myocardial infarction
Dissecting aneurysm
Rupture of esophagus

ABDOMINAL CONDITIONS

Adhesions
Intestinal obstruction
Volvulus
Hernia
Diverticulitis
Cholecystitis/cholelithiasis
Pancreatitis
Appendicitis
Duodenal ulceritis
Cancer
Ovarian tumor
Meckel's diverticulum

VASCULAR CAUSES

Mesenteric embolus or thrombosis
Ruptured or leaking abdominal aneurysm

Differential for acute dyspnea

CARDIAC CAUSES

Atrial fibrillation
Myocardial ischemia
Paroxysmal atrial tachycardia
Bradycardia
Bacterial endocarditis
Acute pulmonary edema
Acute myocarditis
Pericarditis
Valvular disease

PULMONARY CAUSES

Pneumonia
Pulmonary embolism
Pleural effusion
Pneumothorax
Drug reaction
Acute bronchitis
Acute bronchospasm
Aspiration
Cerebrovascular accident
Fat embolism
Noncardiogenic pulmonary edema

Differential for chest pain

CARDIOVASCULAR CAUSES

Myocardial ischemia or infarction
Pericarditis
Aortic dissection
Aortic regurgitation
Aortic stenosis
Mitral valve prolapse

PLEUROPULMONARY CAUSES

Pneumonia
Tumors
Emboli
Pneumothorax
Idiopathic inflammations
Pleuritis

GASTROINTESTINAL CAUSES

Esophageal reflux
Esophageal spasm
Hiatal hernia
Peptic ulcer disease
Cholecystitis
Gastric ulcers
Pancreatitis
Incarcerated intrathoracic stomach

MUSCULOSKELETAL CAUSES

Muscle strain
Costochondritis
Osteoarthritis of cervical and thoracic spine
Rib fractures
Cancer
Pre-eruptive herpes zoster or post-herpetic pain

EMOTIONAL CAUSES

Anxiety attack
Tension
Hyperventilation

Causes of syncope

FOLLOWING NECK TURNING

Hyperactive carotid sinus
Vertebral artery occlusion by osteophytes

WHEN CONSCIOUSNESS IS LOST WITHOUT WARNING

Arrhythmia

WHEN CONFUSION PERSISTS AFTER AWAKENING

Transient ischemic attack
Seizure

WHEN ACCOMPANIED BY NAUSEA, ANXIETY, FEAR

Myocardial ischemia
Vasovagal reaction

WHEN ACUTE ILLNESS IS PRESENT WITH VOMITING, DIARRHEA, POOR INTAKE

Volume depletion
Hypotension

WHEN BROUGHT ON BY EXERTION

Hypertrophic cardiomyopathy
Aortic stenosis
Subclavian steal
Pulmonary hypertension

WHEN ACCOMPANIED BY HYPOTENSION, BRADYCARDIA

Carotid sinus syndrome
Sick sinus syndrome

Appendices

APPENDIX ONE

STANDARD LAB VALUES

All lab values should be evaluated within the context of the person's health profile. The values that follow are reference ranges only, not "normals." Ranges can vary from lab to lab, so be sure to check with yours. Values may also vary depending on the testing method used.

CBC WITH DIFFERENTIAL

Red blood cell (RBC) count	3.6 – 5.4 million/mm^3
Hemoglobin	14 – 18 gm/dL
Hematocrit	37% – 54% (varies widely)
Mean corpuscular volume (MCV)	87 – 103 microns^3
Mean corpuscular hemoglobin (MCH)	27 – 31 picomoles/RBC
Mean corpuscular hemoglobin concentration (MCHC)	32% – 36%
White blood cell (WBC) count	5,000 – 10,000/mm^3

WBC DIFFERENTIAL

Neutrophil count	Relative: 50% – 70% Absolute: 3,000 – 7,000/mm^3
Eosinophil count	Relative: 1% – 4% Absolute: 50 – 400/mm^3
Basophil count	Relative: 0.5% – 1% Absolute: 25 – 100/mm^3
Monocyte count	Relative: 2% – 8% Absolute: 200 – 600/mm^3
Lymphocyte count	Relative: 20% – 40% Absolute: 1,700 – 3,400/mm^3
Platelet count	150,000 – 450,000/mm^3

CHEMISTRIES (CHEM 7)

Potassium	3.5 – 5.3 mEq/L
Sodium	135 – 145 mEq/L
Chloride	98 – 106 mEq/L
CO_2	23 – 30 mEq/L
Glucose (fasting)	65 – 110 mg/dL
BUN	7 – 18 mg/dL
Creatinine	0.6 – 1.3 mg/dL

CHEMISTRIES

Amylase (serum)	25 – 125 U/L
Bilirubin (serum)	Direct: 0.1 – 0.4 mg/dL Total: up to 1 mg/dL
Calcium	8.5 – 10.5 mg/dL
CK (creatinine kinase)	57 – 150 U/L
CK-MB	0 – 3 ng/ml
Iron (serum)	50 – 150 mcg/dL
Iron binding capacity, total (TIBC)	250 – 370 mcg/dL
Lactate dehydrogenase (serum)	94 – 172 U/L
Lipase (serum)	10 – 140 U/L

Lipids, total (serum)
  Cholesterol, total
  Triglycerides
	450 – 1,000 mg/dL
	120 – 220 mg/dL
	40 – 160 mg/dL

Magnesium	1.5 – 2.5 mEq/L
Osmolality (serum)	280 – 292 mOsm/L
Phosphatase, alkaline (serum)	20 – 90 U/L
Phosphorus	2.5 – 4.5 mg/dL

Protein, total (serum)
  Albumin
  Globulin
	6 – 8 gm/dL
	3.5 – 5.5 gm/dL
	2.3 – 3.5 gm/dL

Transaminase (serum)
  SGOT (AST)
  SGPT (ALAT)
  GGT
	
	8 – 29 U/L
	4 – 36 U/L
	8 – 37 U/L

Uric acid	2.5 – 8 mg/dL

COAGULATION TESTS

Platelet count	150,000 – 450,000/mm^3
Prothrombin time	11 – 16 seconds
Activated partial thromboplastin time	30 – 45 seconds
Thrombin time	10 – 15 seconds
Fibrinogen	200 – 400 mg/dL
Fibrin degradation products	< 10 mcg/ml
Antithrombin III	> 50% of control (plasma)
D-Dimer assay	< 100 mcg/L

URINE

Acetone	Negative
Bilirubin	Negative
Calcium	150 – 300 mg/24 hrs
Creatinine	0.6 – 1.8 gm/24 hrs
Glucose	Negative
Osmolality	200 – 850 mOsm/L
Potassium	40 – 80 mEq/24 hrs
Protein (albumin)	Negative
Sodium	130 – 200 mEq/24 hrs
WBCs	0 – 4/high-powered field
Specific gravity	1.003 – 1.035 (usually between 1.010 – 1.025)

THYROID

TSH (thyroid stimulating hormone)	0.2 – 5.4 mcgU/ml
T_3 (free triiodothyronine)	260 – 480 pg/dL or 4 – 7.4 pmol/L
T_4 (free thyroxine)	0.8 – 2.4 ng/dL or 10.3 – 31 pmol/L

APPENDIX TWO

INTERPRETING ABGs

NORMAL ARTERIAL BLOOD GAS VALUES:

pH	=	7.35 – 7.45
$PaCO_2$	=	35 – 45 mm Hg
HCO_3^-	=	22 – 26 mEq/L
SaO_2	=	95% – 100%

If your patient's ABGs do not fall within normal limits, follow these simple rules to identify the problem:

1. LABEL THE pH

pH < 7.35	=	Acidosis
pH > 7.45	=	Alkalosis

2. FIND THE CAUSE OF THE ACID-BASE IMBALANCE

Evaluate the $PaCO_2$ and HCO_3^- in relation to the pH. Let the label of the pH direct you toward finding the cause.

If the pH is < 7.35 and:	Then the problem is:
$PaCO_2$ is > 45	Respiratory acidosis
HCO_3^- is normal	Uncompensated
or	
HCO_3^- is < 22	Metabolic acidosis
$PaCO_2$ is normal	Uncompensated

If the pH is > 7.45 and:	Then the problem is:
$PaCO_2$ is < 35	Respiratory alkalosis
HCO_3^- is normal	Uncompensated
or	
HCO_3^- is > 26	Metabolic alkalosis
$PaCO_2$ is normal	Uncompensated

3. CHECK FOR COMPENSATION

Perform this step if both the $PaCO_2$ and HCO_3^- are abnormal. If there is complete compensation, the pH will be normal; consider a pH between 7.35 and 7.40 as acidosis, and a pH between 7.40 and 7.45 as alkalosis. With partial compensation, the pH will be outside normal limits.

If the pH is < 7.40 and:	Then there is:
$PaCO_2$ > 45	Respiratory acidosis
HCO_3^- > 26	Compensated
or	
HCO_3^- < 22	Metabolic acidosis
$PaCO_2$ < 35	Compensated

If the pH is > 7.40 and:	Then there is:
$PaCO_2$ < 35	Respiratory alkalosis
HCO_3^- < 22	Compensated
or	
HCO_3^- > 26	Metabolic alkalosis
$PaCO_2$ > 45	Compensated

If your patient's ABG results do not match up with any of the groupings listed here, suspect a mixed acid-base imbalance.

APPENDIX THREE

HEMODYNAMIC PARAMETERS

PARAMETER	FORMULA	NORMAL RANGES
Blood pressure (BP)		$\dfrac{90 - 140}{60 - 90}$ mm Hg
Cardiac index (CI)	CO/BSA (body surface area)	2.5 – 4 L/min/m^2
Cardiac output (CO)	SV x HR	4 – 8 L/min
Central venous pressure (CVP)		2 – 6 mm Hg
Cerebral perfusion pressure (CPP)	MAP – ICP (intracranial pressure)	80 – 100 mm Hg
Coronary artery perfusion pressure (CAPP)	Diastolic BP – PCWP	60 – 80 mm Hg
Ejection fraction (EF)		> 50%
Heart rate (HR)		60 – 100 beats/min
Mean arterial pressure (MAP)	$\dfrac{\text{Systolic BP} + 2\ \text{Diastolic BP}}{3}$	70 – 105 mm Hg

HEMODYNAMIC PARAMETERS **183**

Pulmonary artery diastolic pressure (PAD)		5 – 13 mm Hg
Pulmonary artery mean pressure (PAM)		10 – 20 mm Hg
Pulmonary artery systolic pressure (PAS)		15 – 30 mm Hg
Pulmonary capillary wedge pressure (PCWP)		2 – 12 mm Hg
Pulmonary vascular resistance (PVR)	$\dfrac{\text{PAM} - \text{PCWP}}{\text{CO}} \times 80$	120 – 250 dynes/sec/cm^{-5}
Pulse pressure (PP)	Systolic BP – Diastolic BP	30 – 50 mm Hg
Right atrial pressure (RAP)		2 – 6 mm Hg
Stroke volume (SV)	CO/HR	60 – 130 ml/beat
Systemic vascular resistance (SVR)	$\dfrac{\text{MAP} - \text{RAP}}{\text{CO}} \times 80$	800 – 1,200 dynes/sec/cm^{-5}

NOTE: CVP, RAP, PAD, and PCWP readings reflect preload.
Pulmonary and systemic vascular resistances (PVR and SVR) represent afterload.

APPENDICES

APPENDIX FOUR

CALCULATING DRUG DOSAGES AND DRIP RATES

1. Calculating unit dose medications (oral, parenteral, liquid)

Formula: $\dfrac{\text{ordered dose}}{\text{dose on hand}}$ = dose to give

Example: $\dfrac{30 \text{ mg Inderal ordered}}{20 \text{ mg tabs on hand}}$ = 1.5 tabs to administer

2. Calculating a solution's concentration of drug

Formula: $\dfrac{\text{drug amount}}{\text{volume of IV fluid}}$ = mg/cc (solution concentration)

Example: $\dfrac{50 \text{ mg Nitroprusside}}{250 \text{ cc D}_5\text{W}}$ = 0.2 mg/cc

To change mg to mcg, multiply by 1,000
Example: 0.2 mg x 1,000 = 200 mcg

3. Calculating the rate of an IV drip when you know the dose:

Formula: $\dfrac{\text{dose}}{\text{time}} = \text{rate}$

Example: $\dfrac{1{,}000 \text{ cc}}{8 \text{ hr}} = 125 \text{ cc/hr}$

A. When dosage is ordered in mcg/kg/min (or mg/kg/min):

Formula: $\dfrac{\text{patient's weight} \times \text{dose} \times 60 \text{ min}}{\text{solution concentration} \times 1 \text{ hr}} = \text{rate}$

Example: $\dfrac{80 \text{ kg} \times 3 \text{ mcg/kg/min} \times 60 \text{ min}}{200 \text{ mcg/cc} \times 1 \text{ hr}} = 72 \text{ cc/hr}$

B. When dosage is ordered in mcg/min (or mg/min):

Formula: $\dfrac{\text{dose} \times 60 \text{ min}}{\text{solution concentration} \times 1 \text{ hr}} = \text{rate}$

Example: $\dfrac{10 \text{ mcg/min} \times 60 \text{ min}}{200 \text{ mcg/cc} \times 1 \text{ hr}} = 3 \text{ cc/hr}$

C. When dosage is ordered in mg/hr (or units/hr):

Formula: $\dfrac{\text{dose}}{\text{solution concentration}} = \text{rate}$

Example: $\dfrac{28 \text{ mg/hr}}{0.8 \text{ mg/cc}} = 35 \text{ cc/hr}$

4. Calculating the dose when you know the rate

Formula: rate x time = dose
Example: 125 cc/hr x 8 hr = 1,000 cc

A. For a drip running at mcg/kg/min (or mg/kg/min):

Formula: $\dfrac{\text{rate x solution concentration}}{\text{weight x 60 min}}$ = dose/kg/min

Example: $\dfrac{72 \text{ cc/hr x 200 mcg/cc}}{80 \text{ kg x 60 min}}$ = 3 mcg/kg/min

B. For a drip running at mcg/min (or mg/min):

Formula: $\dfrac{\text{rate x solution concentration}}{60 \text{ min}}$ = dose/min

Example: $\dfrac{3 \text{ cc/hr x 200 mcg/cc}}{60 \text{ min}}$ = 10 mcg/min

C. For a drip running at mg/hr (or units/hr):

Formula: rate x solution concentration = dose
Example: 35 cc/hr x 0.8 mg/cc = 28 mg/hr

Other easy-to-remember formulas

To change °C to °F:

Formula: °C x 1.8 + 32 = °F

Example: 37° C x 1.8 + 32 = 98.6° F

To change pounds to kilograms:

Formula: $\dfrac{\text{weight lb}}{1} \times \dfrac{1 \text{ kg}}{2.2 \text{ lb}} = \text{weight kg}$

Example: $\dfrac{170 \text{ lb}}{1} \times \dfrac{1 \text{ kg}}{2.2 \text{ lb}} = 77.3 \text{ kg}$

APPENDIX FIVE

MEDICATION MONITORING: THERAPEUTIC RANGES AND SERUM DRUG INTERACTIONS

DRUG	THERAPEUTIC RANGE
Digoxin	0.5 – 2 ng/ml
Lithium	0.4 – 1 mEq/L
Lidocaine	1.5 – 6 mcg/ml
Phenobarbital	15 – 40 mcg/ml
Phenytoin	10 – 20 mcg/ml
Quinidine	2 – 6 mcg/ml
Theophylline	10 – 20 mcg/ml
Warfarin	Usually 1 1/2 – 2 times normal prothrombin time (PT) INR: 2 – 3, standard therapy; 2.5 – 3.5, high dose therapy

SERUM DRUG INTERACTIONS

Whenever your patient is receiving medication, make sure you know what other drugs he is taking, both prescription and OTC. If he has to take medications that interact with each other, monitor serum drug levels closely and see that drug dosages are adjusted accordingly. Medications that interact with each other are listed below. Keep in mind that these are examples only; for a complete listing of interacting drugs, refer to a drug reference book.

	EXAMPLES OF INTERACTING DRUGS	EFFECT OF THE DRUG INTERACTION
DIGOXIN	Antacids Kaolin-pectin	Decreased digoxin absorption reduces its serum level.
	Nifedipine Verapamil	Serum digoxin increases.
	Quinidine	Serum digoxin increases twofold.
LITHIUM	Diuretics	Decreased renal clearance of lithium raises its serum level.
LIDOCAINE	Cimetidine	Decreased metabolism of lidocaine raises its serum level.
	Propranolol	Decreased hepatic clearance of lidocaine raises its serum level.
PHENOBARBITAL	Valproic acid	Decreased metabolism of phenobarbital raises its serum level.
PHENYTOIN	Quinidine	Increased metabolism of quinidine lowers its serum level.
	Warfarin	Protein-binding competition increases serum phenytoin.

	EXAMPLES OF INTERACTING DRUGS	**EFFECT OF THE DRUG INTERACTION**
QUINIDINE	Barbiturates	Increased metabolism of quinidine lowers its serum level.
THEOPHYLLINE	Cimetidine Erythromycin	Decreased metabolism of theophylline raises its serum level.
	Propranolol	Decreased renal clearance of theophylline raises its serum level.
TRICYCLIC ANTI-DEPRESSANTS	Barbiturates	Increased metabolism of the antidepressant lowers its serum level.
WARFARIN	Acetaminophen	Anticoagulation effect increases.
	Amiodarone Cimetidine	Anticoagulation effect increases due to decreased breakdown in liver.
	Carbamazepine	Anticoagulation effect decreases due to increased breakdown in liver.
	Thiazide diuretics	Anticoagulation effect decreases due to hemoconcentration of clotting factors.
	Vitamine E	Anticoagulation effect increases due to interference with Vitamin K.

APPENDIX SIX

A GUIDE TO TRANSFUSING BLOOD PRODUCTS

Whole Blood

Consists of red blood cells, platelets, plasma, anticoagulant, and preservative. When stored, it loses clotting factors and releases potassium.

INDICATIONS: To treat acute, massive blood loss, but is rarely given. Instead, crystalloid and colloid solutions, red blood cells, or other blood components are usually given.

CONTRAINDICATIONS: Adequate blood volume, availability of specific component

CROSS MATCHING NECESSARY? Yes, must be ABO identical

METHOD OF ADMINISTRATION: Straight or Y-type administration set with standard blood filter

STANDARD UNIT VOLUME: 400 to 500 ml

RATE OF ADMINISTRATION:
Adult: no more than 4 hours
Child: no more than 4 hours, with the amount of blood infused and the rate of infusion dependent on the child's age, size, and condition

POSSIBLE REACTIONS/COMPLICATIONS:
Hemolytic, febrile, and allergic reactions (ranging from urticaria to anaphylactic shock), circulatory overload,

hyperkalemia due to potassium release, hepatitis, HIV, CMV, and other infectious diseases

From massive transfusion: hypothermia, coagulation disturbances, acid-base imbalance, ammonia intoxication, and citrate toxicity that may cause tingling around the mouth, hypotension, nausea, vomiting, alkalosis, hypokalemia, and cardiac arrhythmias

Red Blood Cells

Prepared by removing up to 90% of the plasma surrounding red blood cells, and adding an anticoagulant-preservative. Various preparations include deglycerolized, leukocyte-depleted, and irradiated red blood cells.

INDICATIONS:
Packed: Blood loss and anemia

Deglycerolized: To prevent febrile reactions from leukocyte antibodies

Leukocyte-depleted: To reduce the risk of febrile, nonhemolytic transfusion reactions

Irradiated: To prevent graft-versus-host disease in immunocompromised patients

CONTRAINDICATIONS: Anemia resulting from nutritional deficiency, such as folic acid, iron, or vitamin B_{12}

CROSS MATCHING NECESSARY? Yes, must be ABO compatible

METHOD OF ADMINISTRATION: Straight or Y-type administration set with standard blood filter

STANDARD UNIT VOLUME: 250 to 350 ml, depending on the amount of anticoagulant-preservative

RATE OF ADMINISTRATION: Up to 4 hours

POSSIBLE REACTIONS/COMPLICATIONS:
Same as for whole blood

Plasma

Separated from red blood cells and frozen within 6 hours after collection. Contains plasma proteins, fibrinogen, and factors V, VIII, and IX, along with water, electrolytes, sugar, proteins, vitamins, minerals, hormones, and antibodies.

INDICATIONS: To increase the level of clotting factors in patients with a demonstrated deficiency, or for a single-factor deficiency when precise product is unavailable or unknown.

CONTRAINDICATIONS: When the specific component is available, or for nutritional supplementation or volume expansion

CROSS MATCHING NECESSARY? Yes, must be ABO compatible

METHOD OF ADMINISTRATION: Straight or Y-type administration set with standard blood filter

STANDARD UNIT VOLUME: 185 to 225 ml

RATE OF ADMINISTRATION: May be infused rapidly—10 to 20 ml over 3 minutes, or slowly if potential for circulatory overload exists.

POSSIBLE REACTIONS/COMPLICATIONS: Infectious diseases, allergic reactions, circulatory overload, hemolytic reactions

Platelet Concentrate

Platelets, centrifuged from plasma.
Three types: random-donor, single-donor, and HLA-matched

INDICATIONS: Bleeding due to a deficiency in platelet function or number. Given prophylactically for platelet counts less than 10,000 to 20,000/microliter, and for signs of bleeding with counts less than 50,000/microliter. Also given for aplastic anemia.

CONTRAINDICATIONS: Immune thrombocytopenic purpura unless there is life-threatening bleeding, bleeding unrelated to decreased or abnormal platelets, extrinsic platelet function disorders such as von Willebrand's disease

CROSS MATCHING NECESSARY? ABO compatibility preferred

METHOD OF ADMINISTRATION: Set with platelet filter

STANDARD UNIT VOLUME: 50 to 70 ml

RATE OF ADMINISTRATION: May be infused rapidly—1 unit in 10 minutes or less; must be infused within 4 hours.

POSSIBLE REACTIONS/COMPLICATIONS: Infectious diseases, and septic, toxic, allergic, or febrile reactions; with repeated random-donor transfusions, HLA-antibody reaction may occur.

Cryoprecipitate and Factor VIII

Cryoprecipitate: Obtained from fresh frozen plasma

Factor VIII: Known as antihemophilic factor (AHF), it's also derived from fresh frozen plasma.

INDICATIONS:
Cryoprecipitate: von Willebrand's disease, hypofibrinogenemia, or factor XIII deficiency

Factor VIII: Factor VIII deficiencies including hemophilia type A

CONTRAINDICATIONS: Undefined coagulation deficiency

CROSS MATCHING NECESSARY? ABO compatibility preferred, following plasma compatibility guidelines

METHOD OF ADMINISTRATION: Check the product insert for filter recommendations.

STANDARD UNIT VOLUME: 5 to 20 ml depending on preparation method

RATE OF ADMINISTRATION: Rapidly—1 to 2 ml/min

POSSIBLE REACTIONS/COMPLICATIONS: Infectious diseases and allergic reactions

Factor II, VII, IX, and X Complex

Freeze-dried preparation made from pooled plasma

INDICATIONS: Hemophilia type B (a factor IX deficiency also known as Christmas disease), congenital factor VII or X deficiency

CONTRAINDICATIONS: Use only with specific factor deficiency.

CROSS MATCHING NECESSARY? No

METHOD OF ADMINISTRATION: IV push through a 170-micron filter needle, or IV drip via component recipient set

STANDARD UNIT VOLUME: See product insert.

RATE OF ADMINISTRATION: 2 to 3 ml/min

POSSIBLE REACTIONS/COMPLICATIONS: Allergic reactions and infectious diseases

Granulocytes

Contains granulocytes with variable amounts of red blood cells, plasma, and usually platelets, although some blood collection centers prepare a platelet-poor product.

INDICATIONS: Antibiotic-resistant neutropenia or congenital white blood cell dysfunction. Given infrequently.

CONTRAINDICATIONS: As prophylaxis for infection, and when more conventional therapies haven't yet been tried

CROSS MATCHING NECESSARY? Must be ABO compatible

METHOD OF ADMINISTRATION: Straight or Y-type administration set with filter

STANDARD UNIT VOLUME:
With platelets: 200 to 400 ml
Without platelets: 100 to 200 ml

RATE OF ADMINISTRATION: Very slowly, approximately 50 ml/hr, for up to 4 hours

POSSIBLE REACTIONS/COMPLICATIONS: Circulatory overload and increased incidence of febrile, nonhemolytic reactions

Albumin

Contains albumin, globulin, and other proteins extracted from plasma. Available in 5% solution, which is osmotically equivalent to plasma, and 25% solution, which is concentrated and hypertonic.

INDICATIONS: Acute liver failure, burns, and hemolytic disease of newborn, as well as volume expansion when crystalloid solutions aren't adequate, including for shock and massive hemorrhage

CONTRAINDICATIONS: To treat nutritional deficiencies. Cannot be used as a plasma substitute as albumin contains no clotting factors.

CROSS MATCHING NECESSARY? No

METHOD OF ADMINISTRATION: May be supplied with a special administration set outfitted with a filter; otherwise, check product insert.

STANDARD UNIT VOLUME:
5% solution: 250 ml and 500 ml
25% solution: 50 ml and 100 ml

RATE OF ADMINISTRATION:
5% solution: 1 to 10 ml/min, or more rapidly if patient is in shock
25% solution: 0.2 to 0.4 ml/min

POSSIBLE REACTIONS/COMPLICATIONS: Circulatory overload, hypertension

Source: Harovas, J., & Anthony, H. H. (1993). Your guide to trouble-free transfusions. *RN, 56*(11), 26.

APPENDIX SEVEN

DIFFERENTIATING CHEST PAIN

CAUSE	LOCATION	QUALITY	DURATION	ASSOCIATED SYMPTOMS	PREDISPOSING FACTORS	RELIEF
ANGINA	Substernal; radiates to arms, shoulders (usually left), neck, jaw, or back	Mild to severe pressure, tightness, burning, or squeezing; onset can be sudden or gradual	20 minutes or less	Diaphoresis, weakness	Exercise, emotional stress, temperature changes	Rest, nitroglycerin
ANXIETY	Can be anywhere	Varies in severity and quality; can be dull, sharp, or heavy; onset is sudden	20 minutes or less	Palpitations, dyspnea, sweating, shakes, choking or smothering feeling, nausea, dry mouth	Emotional stress	Rest, anti-anxiety agents

DIFFERENTIATING CHEST PAIN   199

AORTIC DISSECTION	Anterior chest, shoulder, or substernum; radiates to abdomen, back, or legs; location shifts as dissection progresses	Severe stabbing, ripping, or tearing; onset is sudden	Constant	Syncope, confusion, diaphoresis, diminished peripheral pulses	Hypertension, Marfan's syndrome	Narcotics, surgery
BILIARY COLIC	Lower chest around right rib margin; radiates to back	Mild to severe squeezing or tightness; onset is often gradual	Intermittent	Fever, nausea, vomiting	Eating, especially high-fat meals	IV analgesics, surgery
COSTOCHONDRITIS	Rib cage or sternum; confined to one area	Sharp, stabbing pain, often worse on inspiration; onset is sudden	Intermittent	Tenderness over site of pain	Trauma, viral infection	Oral analgesics, steroids
ESOPHAGEAL REFLUX	Epigastrium	Mild to severe burning or gnawing with sudden onset	Intermittent	Acidic taste in mouth	Smoking, alcohol, caffeine, foods high in fat or acid, hiatal hernia	Antacids

(Continued)

APPENDICES

DIFFERENTIATING CHEST PAIN (continued)

CAUSE	LOCATION	QUALITY	DURATION	ASSOCIATED SYMPTOMS	PREDISPOSING FACTORS	RELIEF
ESOPHAGEAL SPASM	Substernal; radiates to left shoulder, chest, or arms	Dull pressure, tightness, or burning; onset is sudden; pain increases in recumbent position	Intermittent		Eating hot, cold, spicy, or acidic foods	Antacids, nitroglycerin
MYOCARDIAL INFARCTION	Substernal; radiates to arms (especially left), neck, jaw, or back	Heavy pressure or burning sensation; constriction varies in severity; onset can be gradual or sudden	Constant	Diaphoresis, pallor, nausea, vomiting, extreme anxiety	Anxiety, exercise, stress, temperature changes, overeating	Nitroglycerin, morphine, thrombolytics
PERICARDITIS	Substernal; radiates to shoulders, neck, or arms	Sharp stabbing pain; increases with inspiration, also aggravated by coughing, swallowing, or recumbent position	Constant	Fever, shallow respirations	Cardiac injury, trauma, infection, uremia, lupus	Oral analgesics, steroids, antibiotics

DIFFERENTIATING CHEST PAIN 201

PLEURISY	Confined to one side of chest	Sharp, knifelike pain; eases with sitting up	Intermittent	Low-grade fever, pleural friction rub	Respiratory infection	Oral analgesics
PNEUMOTHORAX	Confined to one side of chest	Sudden sharp or tearing pain; can be mild or severe	Constant	Dyspnea, cyanosis, tachycardia, diminished breath sounds and chest expansion on affected side	Chest trauma, Marfan's syndrome, growth spurt in adolescent male	Chest tube
PULMONARY EMBOLUS	Substernal; may radiate to shoulder	Varies, may be little to mild pain or severe and sharp; onset is sudden	Varies, can be constant or intermittent	Dyspnea, cyanosis, tachycardia, diaphoresis, hemoptysis, shallow rapid respirations, extreme anxiety	Bed rest, trauma, surgery, acute MI, pregnancy, atrial fibrillation	Morphine, thrombolytics

Source: Merkley, K. (1994). Assessing chest pain. *RN, 57*(6), 58.

APPENDICES

APPENDIX EIGHT

SHOCK: SIGNS AND SYMPTOMS

	HYPOVOLEMIC OR TRAUMATIC SHOCK				EARLY SEPTIC SHOCK	LATE SEPTIC SHOCK	NEUROGENIC SHOCK	CARDIOGENIC SHOCK
	CLASS I	CLASS II	CLASS III	CLASS IV				
BLOOD LOSS (%)	< 15	15–30	30–40	> 40				
BLOOD LOSS (ml)	Up to 750	750–1,500	1,500–2,000	> 2,000				
NEURO	Normal or anxious and restless	Anxious and restless or increasingly lethargic	Agitated, confused	Unresponsive	Mildly confused	Unresponsive	Anxious, restless	Anxious, confused
BLOOD PRESSURE	Normal	Normal	Symptomatic hypotension	Symptomatic hypotension	Low or normal	Symptomatic hypotension	Symptomatic hypotension	Symptomatic hypotension
HEART RATE	< 100	100–120	120–140	> 140	Increased	Increased	Bradycardia	Increased
RESPIRATORY RATE	14–20	20–30	30–40	30–40 or more	Increased	Decreased	Increased	Increased
TEMPERATURE	Normal	Normal	Normal	Normal	Increased	Decreased	Decreased	Low or normal

SHOCK: SIGNS AND SYMPTOMS

CARDIAC OUTPUT	Normal	Decreased	Decreased	Decreased	Increased	Decreased	Decreased	Decreased
CENTRAL VENOUS PRESSURE	Normal	Low normal	Decreased	Decreased	No change	Decreased	Decreased	Increased
PULMONARY ARTERY WEDGE PRESSURE (PAWP)	Normal	Low normal	Decreased	Decreased	Decreased	Decreased	Decreased	Increased
SYSTEMIC VASCULAR RESISTANCE	Normal	High normal	Increased	Increased	Decreased	Increased	Decreased	Increased
SKIN	Pink, cool Capillary refill time (CRT): < 3 seconds	Pale, cool CRT: 3–4 seconds	Pale, cold, moist CRT: > 3 seconds	Pale, cold, cyanotic, mottled CRT: > 3 seconds	Pink, warm, dry	Pale, cold, cyanotic, mottled	Pink, warm, dry	Pale, cold
GASTROINTESTINAL	Normal	Decreased motility	Paralytic ileus	Paralytic ileus	Decrease motility	Paralytic ileus	Paralytic ileus	Necrosis of the intestinal mucosa
RENAL— URINE OUTPUT (ml/hr)	> 30	20–30	5–15	< 5	5 – 15	< 5	Incontinence Atonic bladder	5 – 15

APPENDIX NINE

ELECTROLYTE IMBALANCES: SIGNS AND SYMPTOMS

Potassium imbalances

HYPERKALEMIA	HYPOKALEMIA
Apathy	Abdominal distention
Cardiac arrhythmias (first-degree heart block, ventricular fibrillation, asystole)	Anorexia
	Cardiac arrhythmias
Confusion	Confusion
Cramping	Constipation
Decreased deep tendon reflexes	EKG changes
Diarrhea	Glucose intolerance
EKG changes	Hypoventilation
Irritability	Lethargy
Muscle weakness	Muscle cramps
Nausea	Nausea
Paresthesia	Paralytic ileus
Restlessness	Weakness
Slurred speech	

Calcium and phosphorous imbalances

HYPOCALCEMIA/HYPERPHOSPHATEMIA	HYPERCALCEMIA	HYPOPHOSPHATEMIA
Altered mental status	Agitation	Altered level of consciousness
Bronchospasm	Anorexia	Anorexia
Cardiac arrhythmias	Bone pain	Bone and muscle pain
Carpal and pedal spasm	Coma	Coma
Chvostek's sign—facial muscle spasm on tapping the area over the facial nerve	Confusion	Confusion
Cramping in the extremities	Constipation	Decreased urine phosphorus, bicarbonate, and hydrogen
Fatigue	Heart block	Elevated urine calcium
Hyperreflexia	Hyporeflexia	Frequent fractures
Laryngospasm	Lethargy	Memory loss
Numbness, tingling, or twitching in the extremities	Nausea	Neuromuscular irritability
Paresthesia around the mouth	Personality changes	Seizures
Prolonged QT interval	Polyuria	Tremors
Seizures	Shortened QT interval	
Stridor	Thirst	
Tetany	Ventricular arrhythmias	
Trousseau's sign—carpal spasm on compression of the upper arm with a blood pressure cuff	Vomiting	
	Weakness	

ELECTROLYTE IMBALANCES: SIGNS AND SYMPTOMS

Magnesium imbalances

HYPOMAGNESEMIA	HYPERMAGNESEMIA
Ataxia	Cardiac arrest
Cardiac arrhythmias	Coma
Coma	Drowsiness
Double vision	Flushing
Dysphagia	Heart block
Muscle fasciculation	Hypotension
Nystagmus	Nausea
Seizures	Reduced deep tendon reflexes
Toxic reaction to digitalis	Respiratory depression
Tremors	Vomiting
Vertigo	Weakness
Also: signs and symptoms of hypokalemia and hypocalcemia	

Sodium and chloride imbalances

HYPONATREMIA Serum sodium < 135 mEq/L	HYPERNATREMIA Serum sodium > 145 mEq/L	HYPOCHLOREMIA Serum chloride < 95 mEq/L	HYPERCHLOREMIA Serum chloride > 106 mEq/L
Abdominal cramping	Coma	*The same signs/symptoms as hyponatremia plus:*	*The same signs/symptoms as hypernatremia plus:*
Anorexia	Confusion	Muscle weakness	Signs/symptoms of metabolic acidosis:
Coma	Disorientation	Respiratory arrest	Lethargy, weakness, confusion, and deep labored breathing
Confusion	Fatigue	Slow, shallow respirations	
Dependent edema	Flushed skin	Tetany	
Disorientation	Lethargy	Twitching	
Dizziness	Low grade fever		
Headache	Muscle weakness		
Hypertension	Restlessness		
Lethargy	Seizures		
Nausea			
Postural hypotension			
Restlessness			
Seizures			
Tachycardia			
Vomiting			
Weight gain			

APPENDIX TEN

RECOGNIZING ENDOCRINE EMERGENCIES

Hyperglycemia

DIABETIC KETOACIDOSIS (DKA)
Causes include: Undiagnosed diabetes mellitus; uncontrolled Type I (insulin-dependent) diabetes; Type I diabetes in a patient who is severely stressed (trauma, surgery, infection), omits an insulin dose, or takes an inadequate dose

HYPERGLYCEMIC HYPEROSMOLAR NONKETOTIC SYNDROME (HHNS)
Causes include: Pneumonia and other infections in elderly patients or patients with Type II (non-insulin-dependent) diabetes; total parenteral nutrition, peritoneal dialysis, or hemodialysis; steriods, furosemide, thiazides, propranolol, phenytoin; Cushing's syndrome, chronic renal failure, thyrotoxicosis

Classic signs and symptoms

DKA *versus*	HHNS
Hyperglycemia Blood sugar > 250 mg/dL	Hyperglycemia Blood sugar > 600 mg/dL
Lack of insulin results in the accelerated breakdown of fat, leading to ketosis	Low insulin prevents the breakdown of fat, so no (or low) ketosis occurs
Serum osmolality: 300–350 mOsm/L	Serum osmolality: > 350 mOsm/L
pH < 7.38	pH usually normal, but can be slightly elevated
Elevated serum ketones	Serum ketones normal or slightly elevated
Elevated BUN and creatinine	Elevated BUN and creatinine
Hyperkalemia	Normal potassium
Urine acetone positive	Urine acetone negative
Dehydration	Dehydration
Dry, flushed skin	Dry, flushed skin
Hypotension, tachycardia	Hypotension, tachycardia
Kussmaul's respirations (rapid, deep breathing)	Rapid, shallow respirations
Polyuria, polydipsia, polyphagia	Polyuria, polydipsia, polyphagia
Abdominal pain, nausea, and vomiting	GI symptoms are less severe
Acetone breath	No acetone smell to breath
Mental status changes, from lethargy to coma, related to acidosis	Mental status changes, including lethargy and symptoms of hypovolemia, related to dehydration

Hypoglycemia

Causes include: Overdose of insulin or other hypoglycemic agent; exercise in patients with diabetes mellitus; uncontrolled Type I diabetes; acute alcohol intoxication; malnutrition in renal failure patients; severe liver disease; missed, delayed, or inadequate meal or snack

Classic signs and symptoms

Blood sugar < 70 mg/dL

MILD HYPOGLYCEMIA	MODERATE HYPOGLYCEMIA	SEVERE HYPOGLYCEMIA
Alert, headache	Mild confusion	Disoriented
Irritable	Blurred vision	Seizures, coma
Shakiness	Tremors	Hyperreflexia
Paresthesias		
Hunger		
Tachycardia	Tachycardia	Tachycardia
Normal respiratory rate	Increased respiratory rate	Slow respiratory rate
Pallor	Pallor	Pallor
Cold, clammy skin	Sweaty	Diaphoresis

Keep in mind that hypoglycemia doesn't necessarily start off mild and progress from there. A patient may suddenly develop moderate or severe hypoglycemia or have symptoms of all three. Expect to occasionally encounter unusual symptoms, such as yawning and numbness around the mouth. Also remember that beta blockers can mask adrenergic symptoms.

ADH-Related Conditions

DIABETES INSIPIDUS (DI)
Causes include: Skull fracture; phenytoin; neuro surgery or trauma to the pituitary; cerebral vascular accident (CVA) or aneurysm

SYNDROME OF INAPPROPRIATE ANTIDIURETIC HORMONE (SIADH)
Causes include: Antidiuretic hormone (ADH) secreting tumors (e.g., oat cell of lung, prostate cancer); brain trauma or surgery; viral pneumonia

Classic signs and symptoms

DI *versus*	SIADH
Decreased ADH, kidneys let go of water	Increased ADH, kidneys hang on to water
Sodium > 145 mEq/L (hypernatremic)	Sodium < 135 mEq/L (hyponatremic)
Serum osmolality > 295 mOsm/L	Serum osmolality < 275 mOsm/L
Increased urination (6–24 L/day) —Color: clear —Specific gravity: 1.001–1.005	Decreased or normal urination —Color: dark —Specific gravity: 1.030 or more
Polydipsia	
Complication: severe dehydration	Complication: seizures

Thyroid Disorders

HYPERTHYROIDISM
Causes include: Autoimmune diseases (Graves' disease); toxic nodular goiter; tumors (adenomas, carcinomas); thyroid hormones (levothyroxine); radiation; viral infection

HYPOTHYROIDISM
Causes include: Autoimmune diseases (Hashimoto's disease); diffuse nontoxic goiter; surgical removal of thyroid tissue; iodine deficiency; failure of the gland to produce, or the body to respond to, thyroid hormones

Classic signs and symptoms

HYPERTHYROIDISM *versus*	HYPOTHYROIDISM
Increased T3 and T4	Decreased T3 and T4
Decreased TSH	Increased TSH
Nervousness, inability to sit still	Apathy, slow mental function, generalized fatigue
Fine hand tremors, hyperreflexia	Slow muscle movement
Stare, bulging eyes	Drooping lids, puffy eyes, abbreviated eyebrows
Heat intolerance	Cold intolerance
Tachycardia	Bradycardia
Widening pulse pressure	Normal pulse pressure
Hypertension	Hypotension
Smooth, flushed, moist skin	Coarse, cool, dry skin
	Nonpitting edema (myxedema)
Weight loss	Weight gain
Frequent bowel movements	Constipation
Light menses	Heavy menses

HYPERTHYROIDISM *versus* **HYPOTHYROIDISM**

Life-threatening manifestations:

Thyroid storm—which can be triggered by trauma and stress—characterized by:
  Very high fever
  Lethal arrhythmias
  Severe hypertension
  Worsening of classic signs

Myxedema coma—the severest level of hypothyroidism—characterized by:
  Decreased level of consciousness
  Hypothermia
  Hypotension
  Severe electrolyte imbalance
  Respiratory depression

APPENDIX ELEVEN

CLASSIFYING BURNS

The American Burn Association categorizes burns based on depth of tissue destruction, total body surface area (TBSA) affected, age, cause of the injury, body parts affected, preexisting disease, and trauma. Here are the specific criteria for each category:

MINOR BURN INJURY

Burns of less than 15% of TBSA in adults or less than 10% TBSA in children or the elderly, with less than 2% full-thickness injury.

Minor burns do not involve special care areas like the face, eyes, ears, hands, feet, or perineum.

MODERATE BURN INJURY

Mixed partial- and full-thickness burns of 15% to 25% TBSA in adolescents and young adults; 10%–20% in children under age 10 and adults over age 40.

Full-thickness burns of less than 10% TBSA not involving special care areas.

MAJOR BURN INJURY

All burn injuries totaling more than 25% TBSA in adolescents and young adults; those involving more than 20% TBSA in children under 10 and adults over 40.

Full-thickness burns of 10% TBSA or greater.

All burns involving the hands, feet, face, eyes, ears, and perineum that are likely to result in either functional or cosmetic impairment.

All inhalation injuries, high-voltage electrical injuries, or burns complicated by fractures or other major trauma.

Burns that occur in high risk patients, such as those with diabetes, heart disease, or renal disorders.

Source: American Burn Association. (1984). *Guidelines for service standards and severity classifications in the treatment of burn injury.* 625 N. Michigan Ave., Chicago, IL 60611.

APPENDIX TWELVE

A GUIDE TO RELIGIOUS PRACTICES

SERVICES; SACRAMENTAL SYSTEM	DIETARY REGULATIONS	RELIGIOUS LITERATURE; ROLE OF PRAYER; SPIRITUAL LEADER	BELIEFS ABOUT ILLNESS, DEATH; RITES ASSOCIATED WITH DEATH	BELIEFS ABOUT MEDICAL PRACTICES
Most Protestant denominations				
Sunday services; Christmas and Easter celebrated	None	Bible	Illness a natural part of life	Abortion allowed under certain circumstances
		Private prayer important	Medical treatment accepted	Euthanasia generally disapproved
Two sacraments; Baptism and Lord's supper		Minister	Belief in afterlife	Blood transfusions allowed
			Burial usual; cremation permitted	Autopsy allowed

Roman Catholicism

Principal services on Sunday, six holy days; also daily services	Food intake limited on Ash Wednesday and Good Friday for those between ages 21 and 59	Bible, Missal, prayer books, devotional pamphlets	Illness a natural part of life
Seven sacraments including Baptism, Anointing of the Sick (for every seriously ill patient), and Holy Eucharist (given at patient's request)	Meat not eaten on Fridays of Lent	Private prayer important	Medical treatment accepted
		Priest	Belief in afterlife
			Burial usual; cremation permitted
			Abortion allowed only indirectly, such as during removal of cancerous uterus, to save life of mother
			Euthanasia not allowed
			Blood transfusions allowed
			Autopsy allowed

A GUIDE TO RELIGIOUS PRACTICES

SERVICES; SACRAMENTAL SYSTEM	DIETARY REGULATIONS	RELIGIOUS LITERATURE; ROLE OF PRAYER; SPIRITUAL LEADER	BELIEFS ABOUT ILLNESS, DEATH; RITES ASSOCIATED WITH DEATH	BELIEFS ABOUT MEDICAL PRACTICES
Judaism—Orthodox				
Principal services on Friday at sundown, with Sabbath observed until sundown Saturday; 13 holy days (including five fast days); also daily services	No pork or shellfish, no meat in combination with dairy products; only meat obtained by ritual slaughter permitted	Torah, Talmud, prayer books	Illness a natural part of life	Abortion allowed only if mother in serious danger physically or mentally
	Use of separate dishes/utensils for meat and milk products	Private prayer frequent; special prayers for the sick	Medical procedures avoided on Sabbath if possible	Euthanasia not allowed
Two sacraments: Circumcision and Taharah (washing of body after death)		Rabbi	Belief in immortality of human spirit	Blood transfusions allowed
	Unleavened bread eaten at Passover		Burial as soon as possible after death	Autopsy allowed in some cases

Judaism—Reformed

Services on Friday at sundown, with Sabbath observed until sundown Saturday; nine holy days (including one fast day, Yom Kippur)	Traditional dietary laws followed, but less rigidly	Torah, prayer books	Illness a natural part of life	Abortion allowed
		Private prayer frequent; special prayers for the sick	Medical treatment accepted	Euthanasia not allowed
				Blood transfusions allowed
		Rabbi	Belief in immortality of human spirit	
One sacrament: Circumcision			Burial as soon as possible after death	Autopsy allowed

A GUIDE TO RELIGIOUS PRACTICES

Native American

SERVICES; SACRAMENTAL SYSTEM	DIETARY REGULATIONS	RELIGIOUS LITERATURE; ROLE OF PRAYER; SPIRITUAL LEADER	BELIEFS ABOUT ILLNESS, DEATH; RITES ASSOCIATED WITH DEATH	BELIEFS ABOUT MEDICAL PRACTICES
No regular, formal services or sacraments	None	Prayers chanted; families will hold healing ceremonies or "sings" if space provided	Illness possibly a punishment for bad thoughts or deeds, or caused by spirits	Abortion: no official position, but strong reverence for life
Religious practices include dances, wearing of amulets, use of psychotropic drugs such as peyote	Certain foods, such as cornmeal, believed to have therapeutic properties	Shaman or medicine man	Medical treatment accepted; family may strongly influence patient's decisions	Euthanasia: no official position
			Belief in afterlife	Blood transfusions allowed
			Varying burial practices	Autopsy: no official position

Hinduism

Holy days such as Purnima (day of full moon) celebrated	Some sects vegetarian	Devotional pamphlets	Abortion: no official position, but strong reverence for life
		Private prayer, meditation important	Illness possibly a punishment; faced stoically
Extensive ceremonial system focused on events such as marriage		Priest	Medical treatment generally accepted; faith healing practiced by some sects	Euthanasia not allowed
			Belief in reincarnation	Blood transfusions allowed
			Cremation usual	Autopsy not allowed

A GUIDE TO RELIGIOUS PRACTICES

SERVICES; SACRAMENTAL SYSTEM	DIETARY REGULATIONS	RELIGIOUS LITERATURE; ROLE OF PRAYER; SPIRITUAL LEADER	BELIEFS ABOUT ILLNESS, DEATH; RITES ASSOCIATED WITH DEATH	BELIEFS ABOUT MEDICAL PRACTICES
Buddhism				
Eleven holy days celebrated	Primarily vegetarian	Prayer books Prayer important Priest	Illness possibly a result of sin in previous life Medical treatment accepted; family members may want to assist in care Belief in afterlife Burial or cremation permitted	Abortion; no official position, but strong reverence for life Euthanasia allowed under some circumstances Blood transfusions allowed Autopsy allowed

Islam

Weekly service at noon on Friday	No pork	Qur'an	Suffering predestined; necessity of stoicism	Abortion prohibited or limited by some sects
Feasts such as Eid EL Fitr (Breaking of Fast) and Eid EL Adha celebrated; Lailat AL Qadr (Night of Power) observed	Daytime fasting during Ramaden, ninth month of Islamic lunar calendar	Private prayer five times a day	Medical treatment generally accepted	Euthanasia not allowed
		No organized priesthood; Imam chief officer in mosque	Belief in afterlife	Blood transfusions allowed
No sacramental system			Burial as soon as possible after death	Autopsy allowed for medical or legal reasons

Source: Di Meo, E. (1991). Rx for spiritual distress. *RN, 54*(3), 22.

Bibliography

Abrams, W. B., Beers, M. H., & Berkow, R. (Eds.). (1995). *The Merck manual of geriatrics* (2nd ed.). Whitehouse Station, NJ: Merck.

Alspach, J. G. (Ed.). (1991). *Core curriculum for critical care nursing* (4th ed.). Philadelphia: W. B. Saunders.

Barker, E. (1994). *Neuroscience nursing.* St. Louis: Mosby.

Bates, B., Bickley, L. S., & Hoekelman, R. A. (1995). *A guide to physical examination and history taking* (6th ed.). Philadelphia: J. B. Lippincott.

Beare, P. G., & Myers, J. L. (Eds.). (1994). *Principles and practice of adult health nursing* (2nd ed.). St. Louis: Mosby.

Black, J. M., & Matassarin-Jacobs, E. (Eds.). (1997). *Medical surgical nursing: Clinical management for continuity of care* (5th ed.). Philadelphia: W. B. Saunders.

Carnevali, D. L., & Patrick, M. (1993). *Gerontological Nursing.* (3rd ed.). Philadelphia: J. B. Lippincott.

Epstein, E. (1994). *Common skin disorders* (4th ed.). Philadelphia: W. B. Saunders.

Feetham, S. L., Meister, S. B., et al. (1993). *The nursing of families: Theory, research, education, practice.* Newbury Park, CA: Sage Publications.

Fischbach, F. T. (1996). *A manual of laboratory & diagnostic tests* (5th ed.). Philadelphia: Lippincott-Raven.

Fitzpatrick, T. B., Eisen, A. Z., et al. (Eds.). (1993). *Dermatology in general medicine* (4th ed.). New York: McGraw-Hill.

Fuller, J., & Schaller-Ayers, J. (1994). *Health assessment: A nursing approach.* (2nd ed.). Philadelphia: J. B. Lippincott.

Hanson, C. (1996). *Delmar's Instant Nursing Assessment: Gerontologic.* Albany, NY: Delmar.

Hickey, J. V. (Ed.). (1997). *The clinical practice of neurological and neurosurgical nursing* (4th ed.). Philadelphia: Lippincott-Raven.

Ignatavicius, D. D., Workman, M. L., & Mishler, M. A. (Eds.). (1995). *Medical-surgical nursing: A nursing process approach* (2nd ed.). Philadelphia: W. B. Saunders.

Isselbacher, K. J., Braunwald, E., et al. (Eds.). (1994). *Harrison's principles of internal medicine.* (13th ed.). New York: McGraw-Hill.

Lookingbill, D. P., & Marks, Jr., J. G. (1993). *Principles of dermatology* (2nd ed.). Philadelphia: W. B. Saunders.

Mims, B. C. (1991). *Interpreting ABGs. RN, 54*(3), 42.

Mims, B. C., Toto, K. H., et al. (1996). *Critical care skills: A clinical handbook.* Philadelphia: W. B. Saunders.

Polaski, A. L., & Tatro, S. E. (1996). *Luckmann's core principles and practice of medical-surgical nursing.* Philadelphia: W. B. Saunders.

Porth, C. M. (1994). *Pathophysiology: Concepts of altered health states* (4th ed.). Philadelphia: J. B. Lippincott.

Robbins, S. L., Cotran, R. S., & Kumar, V. (1994). *Robbins pathologic basis of disease* (5th ed.). Philadelphia: W.B. Saunders.

Ruppert, S. D., Kernicki, J., & Dolan, J. T. (Eds.). (1996). *Dolan's critical care nursing: Clinical management through the nursing process* (2nd ed.). Philadelphia: F. A. Davis.

Sabiston, Jr., D. C. (Ed.). (1991). *Textbook of surgery: The biological basis of modern surgical practice* (14th ed.). Philadelphia: W. B. Saunders.

Sapira, J. D. (1990). *The art and science of bedside diagnosis.* Baltimore: Urban & Schwarzenberg.

Seidel, H. M., Ball, J. W., et al. (1995). *Mosby's guide to physical examination* (3rd ed.). St. Louis: Mosby.

Swartz, M. H. (1994). *Textbook of physical diagnosis: History and examination* (2nd ed.). Philadelphia: W. B. Saunders.

Tilkian, A. G., & Conover, M. B. (1993). *Understanding heart sounds & murmurs with an introduction to lung sounds* (3rd ed.). Philadelphia: W. B. Saunders.

Weber, J. (Ed.). (1996). *Nurses' handbook of health assessment* (3rd ed.). Philadelphia: Lippincott-Raven.

Wilson, R. F. (1992). *Critical care manual: Applied physiology and principles of therapy* (2nd ed.). Philadelphia: F. A. Davis.

ART/PHOTO CREDITS

PAGES

15, 16	Figs. 2-1 to 2-4	Steve Munz
29	Fig. 3-1	Richard Johnson, MD
29	Fig. 3-3	Elizabeth A. Abel, MD
30	Figs. 3-5, 3-6	Katherine Bowers, MD
31-32	Figs. 3-7 to 3-12	Richard Johnson, MD
39	Figs. 4-1, 4-2	Barbara Harmon
40	Fig. 4-3	Michael Reingold
44	Fig. 4-4	Barbara Harmon
46	Fig. 4-5	Barbara Harmon
62-64	Figs. 5-1 to 5-5	Steve Munz
65	Fig. 5-6	Barbara Harmon
74	Fig. 6-1	Barbara Harmon
77, 78, 81	Figs. 6-2 to 6-6	Steve Munz
82	Fig. 6-7	Kevin Somerville
94-95	Fig. 7-1	John Foerster
96	Fig. 7-2	Kevin Somerville
98-99	All figures	John Foerster
115	Fig. 8-1	Photo: PHOTRON Illustration: Kevin Somerville
117	Figs. 8-2, 8-3	PHOTRON
122	Fig. 8-4	John Foerster
125	Fig. 8-5	John Foerster
131	Fig. 9-1	Kevin Somerville
137-138	Figs. 9-2 to 9-5	PHOTRON
148, 152, 155	Figs. 10-1 to 10-5	Gina Urwin

INDEX

A

Abdominal
  conditions, 169
  mapping, 131
  pain, 168, 169
Abducens nerve, 40-41, 47
Abuse, physical, 23
Acoustic nerve, 40-41, 49
Addison's disease, 22
AIDS (Acquired
  Immunodeficiency
  Syndrome), 126
Alcohol
  intake, 23
  intoxication, 76
Allen test, 123
Alopecia, 26
Anemia, 22, 26, 75
Aneurysm, 123
  abdominal, 132-133
  aortic, 91, 118
  femoral, 116
Angina, 99
Anosmia, 43
Aortic
  aneurysm, 91, 118
  insufficiency, 91, 102
  stenosis, 101, 116
Aphasia, 57
  expressive, 57
  receptive, 57
Aphasic patients, 3
Appendicitis, 136
Arcus senilis, 91

Areflexia, 65
Arrhythmia, 91
Arterial
  disease, 111, 112, 119,
    121, 123
  insufficiency, 109, 119
  occlusion, 109
Ascites, 129, 134, 135
Asthma, 72, 85
Asymmetry, 58
Atelectasis, 73, 79, 87
Atherosclerosis, 112, 123
Atopic dermatitis, 24
Atrial gallop, 99
Atrophy, 58
Auscultation, 18

B

Babinski's sign, 65
Bacterial endocarditis, 91
Balance, 60-61
Barrel chest, 72
Basal cell carcinoma, 27
Bell's palsy, 52
Biliary tract disease, 24
Biot's respirations, 76
Blindness, 44
Blood, pressure, 120, 121,
  occult, 141
Borborygmi, 132
Bowel
  obstruction, 129, 130
  sounds, 132
Breast examination, 124

Breath sounds, 83-87
  abnormal, 85-87
    crackles, 85
    mediastinal crunch, 87
    pleural friction rub, 87
    rhonchi, 86
    stridor, 86
    wheezes, 85
  assessment, 82-87
  normal, 84
    bronchial, 84
    bronchovesicular, 84
    vesicular, 84
Bronchitis, 86
Bronchophony, 87
Bronchospasm, 85
Bruits, 120, 121, 122, 123

C

CAGE questionnaire, 5
Cancer, 126, 129
  lung, 26
  renal, 140
  skin, 19, 20, 27, 28
  testicular, 150
Cardiac
  auscultation, 96
  disorders, 91, 92
  rhythms, 105
  surgery, 100
  system, 89
Cardiac system
  cycle, 94-95
  in geriatric patients, 160, 165
  questions to ask, 90
Cardiomyopathy, 99
Cardiopulmonary disease, 87
Cataracts, 45, 163
Cellulitis, 25
Chest
  pain, 170, 171
  symmetry, 73
  trauma, 87
Cheyne-Stokes
  respirations, 75
Cirrhosis of the liver, 26, 129, 134
Clubbing
  fingers, 92
  nails, 26, 32
  toes, 92
Compartment syndrome, 109
Congenital heart disease, 102
Congenital valve disease, 101
Consciousness
  level of, 37, 38
  loss of, 168
Consolidation, 87
Contractures, 58
Coordination, 60-62
COPD (chronic obstructive pulmonary disease), 26, 73, 75, 76, 121
Corneal reflex, 48
Coronary artery disease, 91
Corticospinal disease, 65
Cranial nerves, 35-53
  assessment, 42
  disorders, 52-53
  function, 40-41
Cremasteric reflex, 151
Crohn's disease, 129
Croup, 86
Cullen's sign, 130
Cultural data, 6-7
Cushing's syndrome, 130
Cyanosis, 23
  central, 73
  peripheral, 75

D

De Musset's sign, 91
Dehydration, 25
Dermatitis, 111
Diabetes, 111
Diabetic ketoacidosis, 76
Diaphragmatic excursion, 80
  measuring, 80, 81
Diarrhea, 132
Diverticulitis, 129
Drug intoxication, 76
Dysarthria, 51
Dyspnea, 76, 169, 170

E

Edema, 25, 92, 110
  pulmonary, 85
Egophony, 87
EKG, rhythms, 105
Electrolyte imbalance, 65
Emphysema, 72, 79
Epididymitis, 150
Epiglottis, 86
Epispadias, 149
Erythema, 23
Examination
  physical, 11-18
  inspection, 12-13
Extension, 38, 39
External malleolus, 65
Extraocular nerves (CN III, CN IV, CN VI), 47

F

Facial nerve, 40-41, 48-49
Femoral aneurysm, 116
Fever, 25, 75
Flexion, 38, 39
Funnel chest, 72

G

Gastrointestinal system, 127-141
  abdominal assessment
    contour, 129, 130
    movement, 129, 130
    skin, 129, 130
  auscultation, 131-133
  in geriatric patients, 161, 165
  mapping the abdomen, 131
  palpation, 135-140
    bladder, 140
    deep, 136
    kidneys, 139-140
    light, 135
    liver, 136-137
    rectum, 141
    spleen, 139
  uterus, 140
  percussion, 133-135
  questions to ask, 128, 129
Genitourinary system, 143-157
  female, 152-156
    Bartholin's glands, 154
    clitoris, 153
    introitus, 153
    labia majora, 153
    labia minora, 153
    perineum, 153
    pubic hair, 153
    urethral orifice, 153
  in geriatric patients, 161, 166
  hernia assessment, 154-157
  male genitalia, 147-151
    cremasteric reflex, 151
    glans, 149
    penis, 149
    prepuce, 149
    pubic hair, 149
    scrotum, 150
    shaft, 149
    spermatic cord, 151
    testes, 151
    urinary meatus, 149
    vas deferens, 151
  questions to ask, 146
Geriatric emergencies, 167-172
  differential for
    abdominal pain, 168, 169
    acute dyspnea, 169, 170
    chest pain, 170, 171
    coma, 167
    temporary loss of consciousness, 168
    upper GI pain, 168
  neurological diseases, 167
  neurosurgical conditions, 167
  toxic-metabolic disorders, 167

Geriatric patients, 159-172
  age-related changes by system, 160-161
    cardiovascular, 160
    gastrointestinal, 161
    genitourinary, 161
    musculoskeletal, 160
    neurologic, 160
    respiratory, 160
  physical assessment, 162-166
    cardiovascular, 165
    gastrointestinal, 165
    genitourinary, 166
    hearing, 163
    integumentary, 162
    musculoskeletal, 164
    neurological, 162
    respiratory, 164
    taste and smell, 162
    touch, 163
    vision, 163
GI
  bleeding, 129
  distress, 127
  pain, 168
Glasgow Coma Scale, 38
Glossopharyngeal nerve, 40-41, 50
Glossopharyngeal neuralgia, 53
Gout, 25
Graphesthesia, 68

H

Hair loss, 26
Head nerves, 35-53
Hearing impaired patients, 3
Heart
  failure, 75, 92, 99
  sounds, 97-104
Heart disease, 23, 26
  congenital, 102
Heart sounds
  assessment, 97-105
  click, 100
  pericardial friction rub, 100
  prosthetic valve click, 100
  S_1, 97-99
  S_2, 97-98
  S_3, 97, 99
  S_4, 97, 99
  snap, 100
  technique, 97
Hemianopsia, 44
Hemochromatosis, 22
Hemorrhoids, 141
Hepatic
  failure, 130
  tumor, 133
Hepatitis, 129
Hepatomegaly, 134
Hernia, 130
  femoral, 154-157
  inguinal, 150, 154-156
  scrotal, 157
Herpes, 27, 53
History, medical, 6
Hoarseness, 50
Hodgkin's disease, 126
Homans' sign, 124
Hostile patients, 5
Hydrocele, 150
Hyperactive reflexes, 65
Hypercholesterolemia, 91
Hyperpigmentation, 22
Hyperpnea, 76
Hypertension, 23
  pulmonary, 72
Hyperthyroidism, 25
Hypoalbuminemia, 26
Hypoglossal nerve, 40-41, 51
Hypopigmentation, 22
Hypopnea, 76
Hypospadias, 149
Hypothyroidism, 24, 25
Hypovolemia, 93
Hypoxemia, 92
Hypoxia, 76

I

Ileus, 132
Impetigo, 30
Integumentary system, 19-33
  assessment
    color, 21
    lesions, 27-31
    moisture, 24-26
    temperature, 24-26
    texture, 24-26
  questions to ask, 20
Interviewing, 1-9
  closing the interview, 9
  introductions, 2
  patient profile, 6-9
    biographical data, 6
    cultural data, 6-7
    family history, 9
    past history, 9
    psychosocial data, 7
  techniques, 4-5
  with aphasic patients, 3
  with hearing impaired patients, 3
  with hostile patients, 5
  with psychiatric patients, 5
  with speech impaired patients, 3
  with terminally ill patients, 5
  with visually impaired patients, 3
Intestinal obstruction, 132
Intraperitoneal bleeding, 130

J

Jaundice, 24

K

Kidneys, 134, 139-140
Kussmaul's respirations, 76
Kyphoscoliosis, 73

L

Left ventricular hypertrophy, 93
Leg pain, 109
Leriche's syndrome, 109
Level of consciousness (LOC), 37, 38
Lice, 25
Lingual strength, 51
Lipid disorder, 91
Liver, 133-134
Liver disease, 24, 130
Lower motor neuron disease, 65
Lung cancer, 26
Lung disease, 23
Lymphatic system, 124-126
Lymphoma, 126

M

McBurney's point, 136
Malnutrition, 25
Marfan's syndrome, 91, 102
Melanoma, 28
Meniere's disease, 53
Meningitis, 76
Mental status, 57
Metabolic acidosis, 76
MI (myocardial infarction), 99, 100
Mitral
  insufficiency, 102
  stenosis, 103
  valve insufficiency, 91
  valve prolapse, 100
Multiple sclerosis, 52
Murmurs, 101-104
  diastolic, 102, 103
  grading, 104
  systolic, 101, 102
Muscle strength, 58-59, 60
Muscle tone, 58
  flaccidity, 59
  rigidity, 58
  spasticity, 58

N

Nails, 26, 32
Nerves, 35-53
Nervous system, 55-68
  assessment, 55
    balance, 60-61
    coordination, 60-62
    mental status, 57
    muscle strength, 58, 60
    muscle tone, 58
    reflexes, 62-65
    sensation, 66-68
  disorders, 55
  general inspection, 58
  questions to ask, 56
Neurological
  diseases, 167
  disorders, 75, 76
  examination, 35
Neuromuscular disease, 73
Neurosurgical conditions, 167
Nystagmus, 47, 53

O

Obesity, 93
Occult blood, 141
Ocular defects, 91
Oculomotor nerve, 45-46
Olfactory nerve, 40-43
Optic nerve, 40-41, 43-44
Orchitis, 150

P

Pain, abdominal, 168,
Pallor, 75
Palpation, 14-15
  abdomen, 135-140
  bladder, 140
  capillary refill, 113
  chest wall, 76-78
  deep, 14-15
  female genitalia
    Bartholin's glands, 154
    clitoris, 153
    labia majora, 153
    labia minora, 153
    uterus, 140
  hernia, 154-157
  kidneys, 139-140
  light, 14, 15
  liver, 136-137
  male genitalia
    glans, 149
    shaft, 149
    spermatic cord, 151
    testes, 151
  perineum, 153
  pulses, 113-115
  rectum, 141
  spleen, 139
  temperature, 113, 114
Pancreatitis, 129, 130
Paraurethral glands, 154
Parkinson's disease, 58
Percussion, 16-17
  abdomen, 133-135
  respiratory system, 79
    dullness or flatness, 79
    hyperresonance, 79
    resonance, 79
Pericardial effusion, 93, 121
Pericarditis, 100, 121
Peripheral arterial disease, 116
Peripheral vascular disease, 24, 107
Peripheral vascular system, 107-126
  assessment
    discoloration, 111, 112
    edema, 110, 111, 112
    leg pain, 109
    lymphatic system, 124-126
    ulcers, 112, 113
  questions to ask, 108
Peritoneum, 133
Peritonitis, 132, 135
Pharyngeal paralysis, 50
Physical abuse, 23

Physical exam, 11-18
 auscultation
 inspection
  nutritional status, 12
  overall appearance, 12
  posture and gait, 13
  symmetry, 13
 palpation, 14-15
 percussion, 16-17
Pigeon chest, 72
Pleural effusion, 79, 86, 87
PMI (point of maximum impulse), 92, 93
Pneumonia, 14, 17, 73, 79, 84, 85, 86
Pneumothorax, 72, 73, 77, 79
Polycystic disease, 140
Polycythemia, 23
PQRST mnemonic, 8
Preeclampsia, 65
Pregnancy, 22, 93
Proprioception, 67
Psoriasis, 24, 30
Psychiatric patients, 5
Psychosocial data, 7
Pulmonary
 disease, 72, 84
 edema, 85
 fibrosis, 85
 hypertension, 102
 infarction, 86
Pulmonic stenosis, 101
Pulses, 113-115, 116-118
 brachial, 118, 121
 carotid, 118
 femoral, 116, 117
 pedal, 114
 peripheral, 114, 115
 popliteal, 116, 117
 posterior tibial, 116
 radial, 118
Pupil dilation, 45-46

R

Raynaud's disease, 112
Rectum
 assessment, 140
 palpation, 141
Reflexes, 62-65
 assessment
  Achilles tendon, 64
  biceps, 62
  brachioradialis, 63
  patellar, 64
  triceps tendon, 63
 grading, 65
Renal
 disease, 26
 failure, 150
 infection, 134
Respiratory distress, 69, 73, 75
Respiratory failure, 72, 75
Respiratory system, 69-87
 assessment (*see also breath sounds*)
  breathing, 75, 76
  measuring diaphragmatic excursion, 80, 81
  palpation, 76-78
  shape, 71-73
  skin, 71, 73
  symmetry, 71-73
 in geriatric patients, 160, 164
 questions to ask, 70
Rheumatic heart disease, 101, 102, 103
Right ventricular
 failure, 102
 hypertrophy, 93
Right-sided MI, 93
Romberg test, 61

S

Scabies, 25, 31
Scleroderma, 25
Scoliosis, 60, 72, 73

Scotomas, 44
Sebaceous cysts, 150
Sensation, 66-68
  fine, 67
  graphesthesia, 68
  proprioception, 67
  stereognosis, 68
  superficial pain, 66
  temperature, 66
  vibration, 66-67
Skene's glands, 154
Skin cancer, 19, 20, 27
Snellen chart, 43
Speech impaired patients, 3
Spider angiomas, 130
Spinal accessory nerve, 40-41, 51
Spleen, 134, 139
Splenic infarct, 133
Splinter hemorrhages, 91
Squamous cell carcinoma, 28
Staphylococcal infection, 31
Stenosis
  mitral, 103
  pulmonic, 101
Stenotic valves, 99
Stereognosis, 68
Sternocleidomastoid muscle strength, 51
Stroke, 58, 59
Syncope, 171, 172
Syphilis, 26, 27, 31, 43

T

Tachypnea, 75
Terminally ill patients, 5
Thoracic conditions, 168
Thoracic landmarks, 74
Thrombophlebitis, 112
Thrombosis, 110
Tinea capitis, 26
Tinea versicolor, 22
Tinnitus, 53
Toxic-metabolic disorders, 167
Trapezius muscle strength, 51

Trichotillomania, 26
Tricuspid
  insufficiency, 102
  stenosis, 103
  valve, 100
Trigeminal nerve, 40-41, 48
Trigeminal neuralgia, 52
Trochlear nerve, 40-41, 47
Turgor, 25

U

Ulcerative colitis, 129
Ulcers, 111, 129
Upper motor neuron disease, 65
Uremia, 75

V

Vagus nerve, 40-41, 50
Valve disease, congenital, 101
Varicocele, 151
Varicose veins, 111, 124
Vascular
  insufficiency, 120
  sounds, 132
Venous
  disease, 111, 113, 119
  insufficiency, 109, 119
Ventricular gallop, 99
Vertigo, 53
Visually impaired patients, 3
Vitamin B_{12} deficiency, 43
Vitamin C deficiency, 23
Vitiligo, 22, 30
Vocal cord weakness, 50

W

Weber test, 49
Wilms' tumor, 140
Whispered pectoriloquy, 87

X

Xanthelasmas, 91